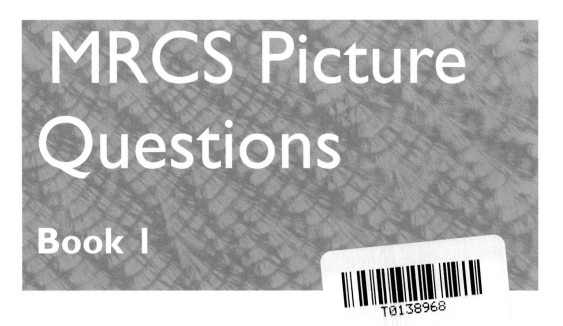

# MRCS Picture Questions

## Book 1

Edited by

**Tjun Tang** MRCS
*Clinical Research Associate
and Honorary Specialist Registrar (Vascular Surgery)
Cambridge University Hospital NHS Foundation Trust*

and

**BV Praveen** MS FRCS (Ed) FRCS (Eng) FRCS (Glasg) FRCS (Ire) FRCS (Gen)
*Consultant Surgeon
Southend Hospital
Honorary Clinical Senior Lecturer
Queen Mary University of London
and Examiner, Intercollegiate MRCS Examination*

Foreword by

**Pradip K Datta** MS FRCS (Ed) FRCS (Eng) FRCS (Glasg) FRCS (Ire)
*Honorary Secretary of RCS (Ed)
and Chief Examiner for MRCS Examinations*

Radcliffe Publishing
Oxford • Seattle

**Radcliffe Publishing Ltd**
18 Marcham Road
Abingdon
Oxon OX14 1AA
United Kingdom

**www.radcliffe-oxford.com**
Electronic catalogue and worldwide online ordering facility.

British Library Cataloguing in Publication Data

A catalogue record for this book is available from the British Library.

ISBN-10: 1 85775 749 1
ISBN-13: 978 1 85775 749 1

Typeset by Advance Typesetting Ltd, Oxfordshire.
Printed and bound by Alden Press (Malaysia).

# Contents

| | |
|---|---|
| **Foreword** | vi |
| **Preface** | vii |
| **List of contributors** | viii |
| **Acknowledgements** | ix |
| **Abbreviations** | x |
| **Section 1: Lumps and bumps** | **1** |
| Pre-auricular dermoid cyst | 3 |
| Incisional hernia | 5 |
| Squamous cell carcinoma | 7 |
| Marjolin's ulcer | 13 |
| Basal cell carcinoma | 15 |
| Malignant melanoma | 17 |
| Port wine stain (naevus vinosus) and strawberry naevus | 23 |
| Shingles | 25 |
| Pilonidal disease | 27 |
| Pyoderma gangrenosum | 29 |
| Erythema ab igne | 31 |
| Xanthelasma | 33 |
| Lipoma | 35 |
| Umbilical hernia | 37 |
| Inguinal and femoral herniae | 39 |
| Liposarcoma | 43 |
| Neurofibromatosis | 45 |
| Clubbing | 47 |
| Sebaceous cysts | 49 |
| Keratoacanthoma | 51 |
| Femoral hernia | 53 |
| Pyogenic granuloma | 55 |
| Rectus sheath haematoma | 57 |
| Ganglion | 61 |
| Hidradenitis suppurativa | 63 |
| Keloid and hypertrophic scars | 65 |

**Section 2: Upper GI tract and hepatobiliary system** — 67

Sengstaken–Blakemore tube — 69
Oesophageal carcinoma — 71
Gastric volvulus — 73
Barrett's oesophagus — 77
Gallstone ileus — 79
Chronic pancreatitis — 81
Acute pancreatitis — 83
Gastric carcinoma causing gastric outlet obstruction — 87
Gallstones — 91
Common bile duct stones — 93
Small bowel obstruction — 95
Meckel's diverticulum — 99
Gastrointestinal stromal tumours (GIST) — 101
Porcelain gallbladder — 103
Small bowel diverticulosis — 105
Pancreatic pseudocyst — 107
Splenomegaly — 109
Subphrenic abscess — 111
Pseudomyxoma peritonei — 113
Free gas under the diaphragm/pneumoperitoneum — 115
CLO test — 117

**Section 3: Vascular** — 119

Acute ischaemia of the lower limb — 121
Charcot's foot — 123
Infected femoral pseudoaneurysm — 125
Ankle brachial pressure index (ABPI) — 127
Ischaemic finger — 129
Varicose veins with ulcer — 131
Popliteal aneurysm — 133
Superficial femoral artery obstruction — 135
Diabetic foot — 137
Carotid stenosis — 141
Below-knee amputation (BKA) — 143
Transmetatarsal amputation — 147
Venous ulceration — 149
Ruptured abdominal aortic aneurysm — 151
Carotid body tumour (chemodectoma) — 153
Lymphoedema — 155
Thoracoscopic sympathectomy — 157
Abdominal aortic aneurysm (AAA) — 159
Superior vena cava syndrome — 163

**Section 4: Head and neck** **167**
Osler–Weber–Rendu disease | 169
Thyroglossal cyst | 171
Parotid tumour (1) and radiotherapy | 173
Lymphadenopathy | 175
Cystic hygroma | 177
Carcinoma of the tongue | 179
Acute lymphadenitis | 181
Parotid tumour (2) | 183
Multinodular goitre | 187
Sialadenitis | 189
Thyroid carcinoma | 191
Branchial cyst | 195

**Section 5: Neurosurgery** **197**
Acute subdural haematoma | 199
Brain abscess | 201
Acute extradural haematoma | 203
Brain metastasis | 205
Carotid atheroma | 207
Traumatic head injury | 209
Pituitary tumour | 211
Depressed skull fracture | 213
Cauda equina syndrome | 215
Subarachnoid haemorrhage | 217
Cervical spine fracture | 219
Chronic subdural haematoma | 221

**Index** **223**

# Foreword

It gives me great pleasure to write a foreword to this book, not least because I have known Mr Praveen ever since his pre-Fellowship days shortly after he came to the UK in the early 1990s. Now, as a Consultant Surgeon in Southend, he has established himself as a good, enthusiastic and committed surgical teacher.

In this day and age surgical teachers are a rare breed. If one was to 'triage' the responsibilities of a surgeon in the NHS, teaching would end up pretty low in the order of priorities – first comes service provision (and quite rightly too), then 'number-crunching' of patients treated to keep managers happy, private practice, research and family. Praveen has been able to strike a superb balance with considerable emphasis on teaching. This book is the outcome of the painstaking collection of clinical material over many years by the two editors, aided by colleagues who have contributed much towards this very worthwhile publication.

Surgical trainees sometimes go from pillar to post in search of good teaching. The MRCS trainees should consider themselves lucky to have this book to prepare for the examination. As an examiner for the MRCS, I can assure the reader that this book comprehensively covers every aspect of Surgery in General including pathology, and answers all questions that can conceivably be asked either in the MCQs or Final Assessment. Some of the material is in such detail that I dare say the book would also be useful for the Higher Surgical Trainee preparing for the Exit FRCS examination.

As a person in the autumn of his surgical career, it gives me immense personal pleasure to see this publication come to fruition – edited by two very committed young teachers, ably supported by several consultants and up and coming young surgeons who are setting out on the road to a surgical vocation. 'A picture is equal to a thousand words' – this adage is exemplified by the excellent pictures in this volume generously contributed by many young surgeons.

In writing this foreword, I must be careful not to stray into making it a 'book review'; that must be somebody else's job. All I can say is that the reader will find the following pages a compelling read. The quality of authorship is such that I will be surprised if other books did not soon emerge from the same stable. I wish the two authors every success.

**Pradip K Datta**
**MS FRCS (Ed), FRCS (Eng),**
**FRCS (Ire), FRCS (Glasg)**
**Honorary Secretary and College Tutor**
**The Royal College of Surgeons of Edinburgh**
**Honorary Consultant Surgeon, Caithness**
**General Hospital, Wick**
***April 2006***

# Preface

It gives us great pleasure to present our book to you. It is designed for candidates sitting both the new intercollegiate MRCS examination as well as the undergraduate clinical examinations in surgery. The method of presentation and topics are drawn from our own experiences during preparation for our examinations. The book provides visual revision material to reinforce core subject matter. The questions are based around a photograph or a set of pictures with each question slightly more difficult than the previous one.

With the new European Working Time Directive and the reduction in doctors' hours, trainees may find it more difficult to be exposed to all the different clinical cases. The MRCS examination requires candidates to acquire knowledge of the presentation and appearance of a wide range of surgical problems and we believe this book allows students and trainees to acquire useful packages of information, not only for examination purposes but also to help them during their clinical practice. The combination of clinical photos and questions is perhaps the best way to revise both the clinical aspects and the subject matter associated with them. It is also believed that seeing clinical cases and reading about them at the same time reinforces knowledge retention.

Case selection is based principally not only upon the editors' experiences but also those of other distinguished clinicians in different sub-specialties. All contributors have been through the rigors of the MRCS examination and several are current intercollegiate MRCS examiners. Typical examination subject material and questions are presented.

We hope you enjoy working your way through this picture book and please do let us have your valued comments. We wish you all the best in your examinations and surgical career.

TT
BVP
*April 2006*

'The conditions necessary for the surgeon are four: first, he should be learned; second, he should be expert; third, he must be ingenious; and fourth, he should learn to adapt himself.'

Guy de Chauliac, 1300–68

# List of contributors

**Iain Au-Yong**
*Specialist Registrar (Radiology)*
*Nottingham Rotation*

**Gerald David**
*Clinical Fellow (General Surgery)*
*James Paget NHS Trust Hospital, Great Yarmouth*

**Stephen Hanna**
*Specialist Registrar (Neurosurgery)*
*Northern Deanery*

**Simon Howarth**
*Honorary Specialist Registrar (Neurosurgery)*
*Addenbrooke's NHS Trust Hospital, Cambridge*

**Aslam Khan**
*Clinical Fellow (General Surgery)*
*James Paget NHS Trust Hospital, Great Yarmouth*

**Kevin Varty**
*Consultant Vascular Surgeon*
*Addenbrooke's NHS Trust Hospital, Cambridge*

**Vamsi Velchuru**
*Clinical Fellow (General Surgery)*
*James Paget NHS Trust Hospital, Great Yarmouth*

# Acknowledgements

**Ashley Brown**
*Clinical Tutor and Consultant Surgeon*
*Southend NHS Trust Hospital, Essex*

**Department of Radiology**
*Southend NHS Trust Hospital, Essex*

**Jonathan Gillard**
*Consultant Neuroradiologist*
*Addenbrooke's NHS Trust Hospital, Cambridge*

**Roger Kittle**
*Medical Illustration Department*
*Southend NHS Trust Hospital, Essex*

**John Latham**
*Consultant Radiologist*
*James Paget NHS Trust Hospital, Great Yarmouth*

**Medical Photography Services**
*James Paget NHS Trust Hospital, Great Yarmouth*

**Saman Perera**
*Consultant Radiologist*
*Southend NHS Trust Hospital, Essex*

**Bruce Smith**
*Consultant Radiologist*
*James Paget NHS Trust Hospital, Great Yarmouth*

**Alphonse Tadross**
*Associate Specialist (General Surgery)*
*James Paget NHS Trust Hospital, Great Yarmouth*

**Geoffrey Waters**
*Consultant Histopathologist*
*Medical Photographer*
*James Paget NHS Trust Hospital, Great Yarmouth*

# Abbreviations

| | |
|---|---|
| AAA | abdominal aortic aneurysm |
| ABC | airways, breathing, circulation |
| ABPI | ankle brachial pressure index |
| ACST | Asymptomatic Carotid Surgery Trial |
| ACTH | adrenocorticotrophic hormone |
| A&E | accident and emergency |
| AF | atrial fibrillation |
| AJC/UICC | American Joint Committee/Union Internationale Contre le Cancer |
| AKA | above-knee amputation |
| ANA | antinuclear antibody |
| ASA | American Society of Anesthesiologists |
| AST | aspartate transaminase |
| ATN | tyrosine-negative oculocutaneous albinism |
| a–v | arteriovenous |
| AVM | arteriovenous malformation |
| AXR | abdominal X-ray |
| BCC | basal cell carcinoma |
| BP | blood pressure |
| BSG | British Society of Gastroenterology |
| CABG | coronary artery bypass graft |
| CBD | common bile duct |
| CF | cystic fibrosis |
| COPD | chronic obstructive pulmonary disease |
| CPP | cerebral perfusion pressure |
| CRP | C-reactive protein |
| CSF | cerebrospinal fluid |
| CT | computerised tomography |
| CTA | computerised tomography angiography |
| CXR | chest X-ray |
| DU | duodenal ulcer |
| DVT | deep vein thrombosis |
| EBV | Epstein–Barr virus |
| ECG | electrocardiogram |
| ECST | European Carotid Surgery Trial |
| EDH | extradural haematoma |
| ELND | elective lymph node dissection |
| ERCP | endoscopic retrograde cholangiopancreatography |
| ESR | erythrocyte sedimentation rate |
| FBC | full blood count |
| FFP | fresh-frozen plasma |
| FGF | fibroblast growth factor |

| | |
|---|---|
| FNA | fine needle aspiration |
| FNAC | fine needle aspiration cytology |
| GB | gallbladder |
| GCS | Glasgow Coma Score |
| GH | growth hormone |
| GI | gastrointestinal |
| GIST | gastrointestinal stromal tumour |
| GORD | gastro-oesophageal reflux disease |
| Hb | haemoglobin |
| HDU | high-dependency unit |
| HPOA | hypertrophic pulmonary osteoarthropathy |
| HS | Hidradenitis suppurativa |
| 5-HT | 5-hydroxytryptamine (serotonin) |
| ICA | internal carotid artery |
| ICP | intracranial pressure |
| IHD | ischaemic heart disease |
| ITU | intensive therapy unit |
| LDH | lactate dehydrogenase |
| ICS | intercostal segment |
| IgG | immunoglobulin G |
| IL-2 | Interleukin-2 |
| ILP | isolated limb perfusion |
| ITP | idiopathic thrombocytopaenic purpura |
| iv | intravenous |
| LA | local anaesthetic |
| LFT | liver function test |
| LVEF | left ventricular ejection fraction |
| MAP | mean arterial pressure |
| MDT | multi-disciplinary team |
| MEN | multiple endocrine neoplasia |
| MI | myocardial infarction |
| MNG | multinodular goitre |
| MODS | multiple organ dysfunction syndrome |
| MRA | magnetic resonance angiography |
| MRI | magnetic resonance imaging |
| NASCET | North American Symptomatic Carotid Endarterectomy Trial |
| NBM | nil by mouth |
| NG | nasogastric |
| NSAID | non-steroidal anti-inflammatory drug |
| OCP | oral contraceptive pill |
| OGD | oesophagogastro duodenoscopy |
| OPSI | opportunist post-splenectomy infection |
| PDS | polydiaxanone suture |
| PE | pulmonary embolism |
| PEG | percutaneous endoscopic gastrostomy |
| PET | positron emission tomography |
| $Po_2$ | partial pressure of oxygen |
| PPI | proton pump inhibitor |
| PR | per rectum |
| PRIND | prolonged reversible ischaemic neurological deficit |
| PRL | prolactin |
| PTA | percutaneous transfemoral angioplasty |
| PTC | percutaneous transhepatic cholangiogram |

| | |
|---|---|
| RBC | red blood cell |
| RCT | randomised controlled trial |
| RTA | road traffic accident |
| SBO | small bowel obstruction |
| SCC | squamous cell carcinoma |
| SFA | superficial femoral artery |
| SFJ | sapheno-femoral junction |
| SIRS | systemic inflammatory response syndrome |
| SLNB | sentinel lymph node biopsy |
| SPF | sun protection factor |
| SPJ | sapheno-popliteal junction |
| SVC | superior vena cava |
| TB | tuberculosis |
| TFT | thyroid function test |
| TIA | transient ischaemic attack |
| TIPSS | transjugular intrahepatic porto-systemic shunting |
| TNM | tumour, node, metastasis |
| TOE | transoesophageal echo |
| TPN | total parenteral nutrition |
| TTE | transthoracic echo |
| USS | ultrasound scan |
| UV | ultraviolet |
| VZV | varicella zoster virus |
| WCC | white cell count |

**To Mummy and Papa for all their love and
support over the years. TT**


**In memory of
MY PARENTS as their
Golden Wedding Anniversary tribute. BVP**

# Section 1

# Lumps and bumps

# Pre-auricular dermoid cyst

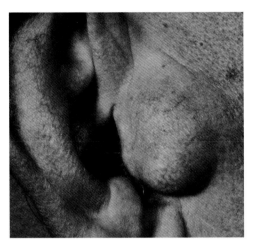

**Figure 1.1**

A 17-year-old boy noticed this lump recently around his right ear. He had sustained an injury to the same area 6 months ago.

## Questions

**Q1** Describe the clinical picture.

**Q2** What is the most likely diagnosis?

**Q3** What is the embryological basis of this condition?

**Q4** How would you treat this condition?

## Answers

**A1** The lump is smooth and hemispherical in the pre-auricular region. There is an associated scar from a previous injury.

**A2** Pre-auricular dermoid cyst. The differential diagnoses should include an unfused embryological auditory tubercle, parotid lump and pre-auricular lymph node.

**A3** A dermoid cyst is a skin-lined cyst deep to the skin. It may be congenital or acquired.
- *Congenital*: due to developmental inclusion of epidermis along lines of fusion of skin dermatomes and therefore found commonly at:
  - medial and lateral ends of the eyebrows
  - midline of the nose (nasal dermoid cysts)
  - midline of the neck and trunk
- *Acquired*: due to forced implantation of skin into subcutaneous tissues following an injury.

**A4** Surgical treatment involves complete excision of the cyst. If congenital, surgical treatment involves complete excision but the full extent of the cyst should be established with suitable radiographic views. This is especially important in midline cysts which may communicate with the CSF, so exclusion of a bony defect is vital before surgery.

## Incisional hernia

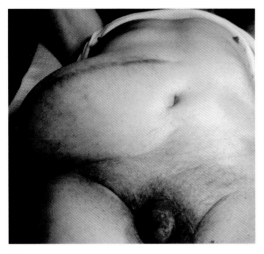

**Figure 1.2**

This patient noticed a non-tender reducible lump under an old scar. It has gradually enlarged over the last few years.

### Questions

Q1  What is it? Define the term.

Q2  What are the potential complications?

Q3  What factors predispose to the development of such an entity?

Q4  What are the treatment options?

Q5  What are the recurrence rates after surgical treatment?

## Answers

 An incisional hernia is the extrusion of peritoneum and abdominal contents through a weak scar or accidental wound on the abdominal wall.

 Potential complications are:
- intestinal obstruction (often intermittent)
- incarceration and strangulation
- skin excoriation
- pain.

 Divide the causes into pre-operative, operative and post-operative factors:
- *pre-operative*: age, immunosuppressed state (renal failure, diabetes, steroid use), obesity, malignancy, malnutrition, abdominal distension from obstruction or ascites; local skin/tissue sepsis, cardiopulmonary disease
- *operative*: technical failure by surgeon – poor incision, poor closure (too small bites or inappropriate suture material, placement of drains through wounds). Also high-risk incisions – lower/upper midline, lateral muscle splitting, subcostal, parastomal and transverse
- *post-operative*: haematoma, infection, necrosis, post-operative atelectasis and chest infection, early exertion.

 There are non-surgical and surgical options.
- *Non-surgical*: consider if the patient is asymptomatic and has multiple co-morbidities, hernia is wide-necked and easily reducible. Methods are:
  - observation
  - use of a corset or truss
  - weight loss and management of risk factors.
- *Surgical*: consider if:
  - symptomatic
  - there is a cometic consideration
  - there are complications of the hernia – irreducibility, obstruction, strangulation, perforation/abscess within hernia sac.
- *Prior to surgery*: optimise cardiorespiratory status and other risk factors, weight loss.
- Give proper counselling regarding recurrence and complications.
- *Surgical principles*: layer-to-layer anatomical repair, mesh repair, keel repair
  - dissect out the hernia sac from surrounding tissues and ensure definition of all bordering tissue to at least 2–3 cm
  - close the defect and then use onlay mesh overlapping normal tissue to allow healing (~3 cm) – superior to suture technique
  - use a layered closure technique with sutures (if no tissue loss)
  - a large hernia may require placement of post-operative drains.
- Laparoscopic repair is presently an option.

 Recurrence varies from 1% to 40%; it is lower with mesh repairs (~10%):
- open anatomical repair: 25–40%
- open mesh repair: 10%
- laparoscopic repair: 7–15%.

# Squamous cell carcinoma

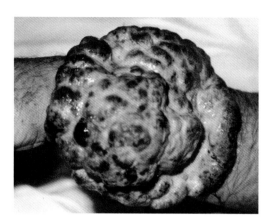

**Figure 1.3**

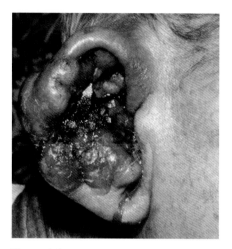

**Figure 1.4**

Figures 1.3 and 1.4 are examples of the same disease affecting different regions of the body.

## Questions

Q1   What is the most likely diagnosis?

Q2   What are the characteristics of skin? Discuss the relevant anatomy/histology.

Q3   What are the modes of presentation of this lesion?

Q4   What are the histological changes in this condition?

Q5   What is the mode of diagnosis?

Q6   What are the treatment modalities?

## Answers

 Squamous cell carcinoma.

 Characteristics of skin are:
- it is the heaviest organ: 16% total body weight and 1.2 to 2.3 m² surface area
- it is composed of epidermis and dermis
- functions include:
  - protection – physical, biological, against UV light, from dehydration
  - regulation of body temperature
  - synthesis of vitamin D with UV absorption
  - sensory.

**Epidermis**
- It is keratinised stratified squamous epithelium.
- Turnover from basal to superficial ranges from 25 to 50 days.
- Specialised structures include sweat glands and hair follicles.
- It is regenerated by the keratinocyte cell lineage: stem cells in the basal layer differentiate as they move outwards.
- It consists of five layers or strata:
  - stratum basale: deepest
  - stratum spinosum
  - stratum granulosum
  - stratum lucidum
  - stratum corneum: surface.

*Stratum basale*
- Single layer of columnar or cuboidal keratinocyte stem cells, which are mitotically active.
- Deepest layer.
- Attached to basement membrane by hemidesmosomes; attached to each other with desmosomes.
- Melanocytes and Merkel cells present.

*Stratum spinosum*
- Several layers of cuboidal, polygonal and slightly flattened cells, with a central euchromatic nucleus; mitotically active.
- Concentrated tonofilaments in the cytoplasm.
- Langerhans cells.
- Projections of melanocytes.
- Psoriasis: skin disorder where excessive cell division leads to increased thickening of strata basale and spinosum.
- Cytoplasm is rich in tonofilaments that terminate with desmosomes in spiny projections, hence 'spinosum' – they hold the cells together and help protect the skin from abrasion.
- Shrinkage of the keratinocytes reveals the spines.

*Stratum granulosum*
- 3 to 5 layers of flattened polygonal cells.
- Cells accumulate keratohyalin granules with phosphorylated his- and cys-rich proteins, hence 'granulosum'.

- Cells also contain lamellar granules which are lipid and protein rich, and are discharged extracellularly to produce a 'cement' that seals the skin to foreign objects and water.
- Most superficial layer in which nuclei are present, but no cell division occurs.

*Stratum lucidum*
- A translucent thin layer of extremely flattened eosinophilic cells.
- Nuclei and organelles are not present.
- Filaments and desmosomes are retained.
- Cells contain eleidin, a transformation product of keratohyalin.

*Stratum corneum*
- Outermost layer.
- Composed of 15 to 20 layers of flattened, non-nucleated, keratinised cells: filled with filamants of keratin.
- Surface cells continuously desquamated.

*Specialised cells*
- *Langerhans cells*:
  - bone marrow-derived monocyte/macrophage cell that is antigen presenting
  - present in all layers, but predominantly in the stratum spinosum
  - pale nuclei, granular cytoplasm, processed
  - increase in number in chronic inflammatory skin diseases.
- *Merkel's cells*:
  - rare in thin skin
  - in the stratum basale
  - contain small dense granules
  - may function as sensory mechanoreceptors or as neuroendocrine cells.
- *Melanocytes*
  - present in the stratum basale
  - pale 'halo' of cytoplasm
  - neural crest
  - produce melanin and pass it on to nearby keratinocytes
  - melanin covers nuclei of keratinocytes
  - skin colour depends on activity of cells, rather than number.

**Dermis**
- Dense irregular connective tissue; type I collagen.
- Networks of elastic fibres, blood vessels, nerves and nerve endings.
- Blood vessels in skin are important in blood temperature and pressure regulation.
- In old age, cross-linking of fibres increases and the number of elastic fibres decreases.
- *Dermal papillae*: interdigitations of the dermis and the epidermis which counteract the shearing force between the two layers – prominent in areas that grip or experience friction, e.g. fingertips, palms, soles of feet.
- *Layers*:
  - *papillary layer* – loose arrangement of cells that forms the dermal papillae, loops of small blood vessels and capillaries, nerve endings
  - *reticular layer* – dense irregular arrangement of cells that forms the bulk of the dermis, with blood vessels and a–v shunts, lymphatics and nerves.

**Hypodermis**
- Loose connective tissue consisting largely of adipose tissue.

- Erythematous, ulcerated, crusting lesion.
- Area of persistent ulceration.
- Hyperkeratotic patch.
- Opaque nodule with or without ulceration.
- Actinic keratosis (a premalignant condition that may develop into squamous cell carcinoma).

**Squamous cell carcinoma-in-situ**
- Full-thickness involvement of the epidermis by atypical and dysplastic cells.
- Features include loss of orderly maturation as cells progress from basal to superficial layers.
- Significant variability in nuclear size, shape, and staining between neighbouring cells.
- Mitoses at higher than expected levels.
- Multinucleation.
- Dyskeratosis, hyperkeratosis, and parakeratosis.
- Bowen disease of the skin and erythroplasia of Queyrat of the penis are clinical expressions of squamous cell carcinoma-in-situ.
- Lesions with features that fall short of full-thickness involvement are characterised as actinic (solar) keratosis.
- Different variants and patterns, such as psoriasiform pattern, atrophic form, verrucous hyperkeratotic type, pigmented type, and Pagetoid variant.

**Invasive squamous cell carcinoma**
- A malignant squamous neoplasm in which the cells have penetrated the epithelial basement membrane and invaded the dermis for a variable distance.
- Cells have abundant eosinophilic-to-organophilic cytoplasm with observable desmosomal bridges between cells.
- The nucleus is enlarged, irregular, and often vesicular.
- The tumour is graded subjectively according to the degree of anaplasia and keratinisation.
- Tumours can be graded as well, moderately, and poorly differentiated.
- Well-differentiated tumours may display abundant organophilic (keratinised) cytoplasm, extracellular squamous pearls, and little nuclear anaplasia.
- Poorly differentiated neoplasms may not be recognisable as squamous in origin, except for the fact that the neoplasms are observed deriving from the epidermis. These lesions tend to have large nuclear-to-cytoplasmic ratios, high degrees of nuclear anaplasia, frequent mitosis, and no observable intracellular or extracellular keratinisation.
- Moderately differentiated SCCs fall somewhere between these two extremes.
- Variants of SCC are named according to their architectural features, including spindle cell type, adenoid type, and verrucous type.

- Punch biopsy.
- Incisional biopsy.
- Excisional biopsy.

- Surgery is the mainstay of treatment of these types of cancer. Wide local excision with a 0.5 cm margin and primary closure is adequate in most cases.

- *Mohs' micrographic surgery*: the surgery is performed using sequential excisions and histological examination of the entire surgical margin. Subsequent excisions are performed only of the areas with persistent disease. The procedure is terminated when no residual disease remains.
- It is recommended that invasive squamous cell carcinoma not be treated with curettage and electro-fulguration, cryotherapy or topical 5-fluorouracil, as it is not possible to be sure of adequacy of removal of the squamous cell carcinoma with these modalities. These are reserved for use only in very special circumstances.
- Risk factors for metastatic disease to regional lymph nodes include primary site tumour greater than 2 cm, depth greater than 6 mm, rapid growth, poorly differentiated tumours, immunocompromised host state, anatomical site (e.g. ear, temple, lip), and perineural invasion.
- A detailed assessment of the regional lymph nodes is done at the initial presentation and at each follow-up visit.
- Nodal dissection is not usually indicated for patients with N0 stage. Monitor these patients, especially for the first 2 years. Rarely, prophylactic radiation to the draining area is considered.
- Lymphadenectomy is indicated when regional lymph nodes are involved.
- If cancer involves the skin or a scar from a previous excision or biopsy, include these areas in the surgical specimen.
- Radiation is reserved for unusual cases.
- Patients who have distal metastatic disease do poorly. Combination surgery, radiation, and chemotherapy may benefit selected patients.

**Your revision notes:**

## Marjolin's ulcer

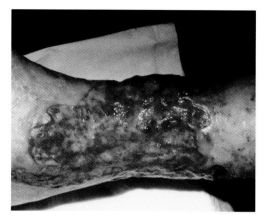

**Figure 1.5**

### Questions

Q1  Describe the lesion.

Q2  What is the most likely diagnosis?

Q3  What are the risk factors for the development of varicose ulcers?

Q4  What is the aetio-pathogenesis of this ulceration?

Q5  What are the other causes of leg ulcers?

Q6  How is this treated?

## Answers

**A1** There is an irregular ulcer involving the gaiter's area of the leg near the medial malleolus with the relevant dimensions. The edge of this ulcer is mostly sloping in nature but appears everted at a few locations. The floor of the ulcer is rather clean and covered by patchy areas of protuberant granulation tissue, possibly exposing the underlying structures. There is no slough or patches of necrosis. The adjacent skin demonstrates chronic changes of venous eczema and lipodermatosclerosis.

**A2** This is a chronic venous ulcer with a possible element of malignant change – squamous cell carcinoma 'Marjolin's ulcer'.

**A3**
- Obesity.
- Varicose veins.
- Prolonged sitting or standing.
- Previous DVT or phlebitis.
- Previous trauma to extremity.
- Pelvic masses.
- Pregnancy.
- Congenital defects in the veins (Klippel–Trénaunay syndrome).
- Age-related loss of support to the veins.

**A4** Chronic venous stasis due to incompetent veins or valves or the perforators, leads to a build up of pressure around the ankle. This leads to lysis of the red blood corpuscles and consequently haemosiderin deposition. The local stagnation and hypoxia perpetuate the 'white cuff' theory by recruiting the neutrophils and macrophages/histiocytes, leading to the build up of an inflammatory cascade. Oxygen free radicals are responsible for the tissue injury. This causes destruction/skin breakdown and tampers with normal healing.

**A5**
- *Arterial disorders*: atherosclerosis, Buerger's disease, polyarteritis nodosa.
- *Small-vessel disease*: diabetes, rheumatoid arthritis, vasculitis, hypertension, sickle cell.
- *Infection*: tuberculosis, Buruli ulcer, mycetoma, syphilis.
- *Neuropathy*: diabetes mellitus, leprosy, syphilis, syringomyelia.
- *Neoplasia*: squamous cell carcinoma, Kaposi's sarcoma, malignant melanoma.
- *Trauma*: direct injury, artefact.
- *Idiopathic*: pyoderma gangrenosum, necrobiosis lipoidica.

**A6**
- Limb elevation.
- Regular cleaning and dressing of the ulcerations.
- Four-layer compression bandage technique.
- If there is venous incompetence causing varicosities, then this is to be dealt with accordingly.
- Skin graft if appropriate (clean area to be grafted and after the surgical treatment to the varicosities).
- Control of co-morbid factors may be a compulsory element.
- Not surprisingly, an amputation may be an end-stage treatment in severe non-salvageable cases.
- If there is an element of a carcinomatous change, then multiple biopsies and further treatment as appropriate are needed.

# Basal cell carcinoma

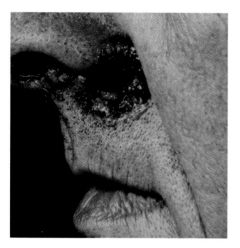

Figure 1.6

## Questions

**Q1** What is the most likely diagnosis?

**Q2** What are the predisposing factors in the development of this condition?

**Q3** At what age and in which sex does this disease characteristically develop?

**Q4** What is the typical body distribution and what are the different forms?

**Q5** What are the various treatment options available?

**Q6** From where are these cells thought to originate?

## Answers

(A1) Rodent ulcer or basal cell carcinoma.

(A2)
- Light skin.
- Sun exposure.
- Exposure to arsenic (used in Fowler's solution – potassium arsenite to treat diverse diseases like psoriasis and asthma).
- Hereditary predispositions include albinism, xeroderma pigmentosa, nevoid basal cell carcinoma syndrome, Rasmussen syndrome and Rombo syndrome.

(A3)
- Affects age group between 40 and 79 years.
- Affects more men than women.

(A4)
- 85% occurs in the head and neck region.
- Nodular 50–54%.
- Superficial 9–11%.
- Cystic 4–8%.
- Pigmented 6%.
- Morpheic 2%.

(A5)
- Surgical excision (in the exam mention about Langer's line and look for previous excision scars before you commit on the incision you will use).
- Radiotherapy: BCC is very radiosensitive; this is probably the treatment of choice for the patient in the picture. Recurrence rate is 8.7%.
- Electrodessication and curettage – for small lesions.
- Mohs' micrographic surgery: good response with recurrence rates as low as 1%. Best choice for certain recurrent BCC and for lesions in canthi, nasolabial folds and post-auricular folds.

(A6) From pluripotent epithelial cells of the basal layer of the epidermis and hair cells.

## Malignant melanoma

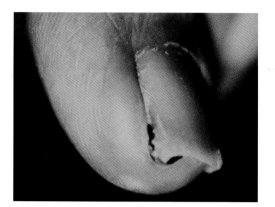

**Figure 1.7**

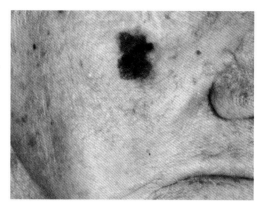

**Figure 1.10**

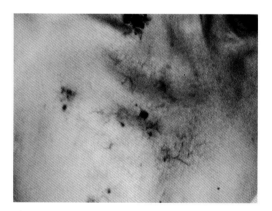

**Figure 1.8**

### Questions

**Q1** What could Figure 1.7 represent?

**Q2** What is the likely diagnosis in Figure 1.8, bearing in mind the diagnosis made for Figure 1.7?

**Q3** What is melanin? Describe its role.

**Q4** What are the aetio-pathogenesis and predisposing factors in the development of this condition? What does Figure 1.9 show?

**Q5** What are the different subtypes? Which subtype is being demonstrated in Figure 1.10?

**Q6** Can you describe any systems that aid in diagnosis of a suspicious skin lesion?

**Q7** What are the stages of tumour progression?

**Q8** What are surrounding lesions?

**Q9** What are the factors assessed on an excision biopsy lesion?

**Q10** What are the systems used to grade this condition? Which gives the better prognosis and why?

**Q11** What are the preventive aspects to be encouraged?

**Q12** What are the treatment options available?

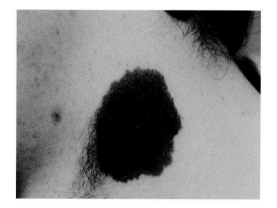

**Figure 1.9**

## Answers

**A1** This picture could represent either a sub-ungual haematoma or a sub-ungual melanoma. The features that would support melanoma will be extensive involvement of peri-ungual skin (Hutchinson's sign).

**A2** Advanced cutaneous melanoma.

**A3** Melanin is a water-insoluble polymer of various compounds derived from the amino acid tyrosine. The synthesis of melanin is catalysed by the enzyme tyrosinase; an inherited lack of tyrosinase activity results in one of the forms of albinism. Tyrosinase is found in only one specialised type of cell, the melanocyte, and in this cell melanin is found in membrane-bound bodies called melanosomes. Melanosomes can be transferred from their site of synthesis in the melanocytes to other cell types. The various hues and degrees of pigmentation found in the skin of human beings are directly related to the number, size, and distribution of melanosomes within the melanocytes and other cells. It is one of two pigments found in human skin and hair and adds brown to skin colour; the other pigment is carotene, which contributes yellow colouring. Besides its role in pigmentation, melanin, which absorbs ultraviolet light, plays a protective role when skin is exposed to the damaging rays of the sun.

**A4** Primary cutaneous melanoma may develop in precursor melanocytic naevi (commonly acquired, congenital, and atypical/dysplastic types), although more than 50% of cases are believed to arise *de novo* without a pre-existing pigmented lesion. Melanoma is multi-factorial and appears to be related to multiple risk factors including:
- presence of a changing mole on the skin
- fair complexion + prominent freckling tendency
- excessive sun exposure and blistering sunburns – classically intermittent high-energy exposure compared to continuous low-energy exposure
- increased number of commonly acquired and dysplastic moles
- family history of melanoma (2–10%).

Figure 1.9 shows Hutchinson's freckle.

**A5**
- Superficial spreading melanoma (SSM).
- Lentigo maligna melanoma (LMM).
- Nodular melanoma (NM).
- Acral lentigous melanoma – sub-ungual belongs to this group; it is more common in dark-skinned individuals.
- Amelanocytic melanoma.

Figure 1.10 shows lentigo maligna melanoma.

**A6** **Glasgow system or MacKie's seven-point checklist:**
*Major (carries two points each):*
- change in size
- irregularity of pigmentation
- irregularity of outline.

*Minor (carries one point each):*
- diameter greater than 6 mm
- inflammation
- oozing or bleeding
- itch or altered sensation.

Needs further evaluation in the presence of one major or if scores reach three.

**American ABCDE system**
A Asymmetry (opposite segments of the lesion are different).
B Border (irregular, resembling coastline with bays and promontories).
C Colour variation.
D Diameter greater than 6 mm.
E Used to be for elevation but now it is meant to be for examination for other lesions.

(A7) Five stages of tumour progression have been suggested:
1 benign melanocytic naevi
2 melanocytic naevi with architectural and cytologic atypia (dysplastic naevi)
3 primary malignant melanoma, radial growth phase
4 primary malignant melanoma, vertical growth phase
5 metastatic malignant melanoma.

(A8) Possible satellite nodules or in-transit metastatic deposits.

(A9) An excisional biopsy with adequate margins is preferred to ascertain the following information:
- assessment of tumour depth (Breslow depth)
- anatomic level of invasion (Clark's level)
- ulceration
- presence of mitoses
- lymphatic/vessel invasion or vascular involvement
- host response (tumour-infiltrating lymphocytes)
- regression
- immunohistochemical staining for lineage (S-100, homatropine methylbromide 45) or proliferation markers (proliferating cell nuclear antigen, Ki67).

(A10) **Clark's classification (level of invasion)**
- *Level I:* lesions involving only the epidermis (*in situ* melanoma); not an invasive lesion.
- *Level II:* invasion of the papillary dermis, but does not reach the papillary–reticular dermal interface.
- *Level III:* invasion fills and expands the papillary dermis, but does not penetrate the reticular dermis.
- *Level IV:* invasion into the reticular dermis but not into the subcutaneous tissue.
- *Level V:* invasion through the reticular dermis into the subcutaneous tissue.

**Breslow (depth) thickness of the lesion**
Tumour thickness, as defined by the Breslow depth, is the most important histological determinant of prognosis and is measured vertically in millimetres from the top of

the granular layer (or base of superficial ulceration) to the deepest point of tumour involvement. Increased tumour thickness confers a higher metastatic potential and a poorer prognosis. The categories are:
- ≤0.75 mm
- 0.76–1.5 mm
- 1.5–4 mm
- ≥4 mm.

Breslow gives the better indication of prognosis. In Clark's levels, the thicknesses of the papillary and reticular dermis vary around the body: both are thin on the face but thick on the back.

 The preventive aspects are:
- adequate clothing
- UV-absorbent screens. Use of a sunscreen with an SPF of at least 15 daily is recommended. Ultraviolet radiation especially in the wavelength range of 320–280 nm is the most carcinogenic, but tumours can also occur in the wavelength range of 250–300 nm. UVC, which is in the range of 280–300 nm, is normally absorbed by ozone. But with the depletion of ozone by chlorofluorocarbons UVC may also gain importance in the production of skin malignancies
- avoiding sunbathing and tanning salons. UV rays from artificial sources such as tanning beds and sunlamps are just as dangerous as those from the sun
- avoiding sun exposure particularly for those patients at risk (albinism, xeroderma pigmentosa, etc)
- systemic enhancement of skin resistance
- local or systemic carotenoids (carotene, retinol, retinoids) prevent malignant transformations. Systemic retinoids are more effective
- public education/regular skin check up is vital for early detection and regular follow-up.

 **Surgical management**
- Excision margin based on histological confirmation of tumour-free margins:
  - for melanoma *in situ*: 0.5 cm margins
  - melanoma with Breslow thickness <2 mm: 1.0 cm margins
  - melanoma with Breslow thickness > or equal to 2.0 mm: 2.0 cm margins.
- Melanomas near a vital structure may require a reduced margin.
- Aggressive histological features may warrant a wider margin.
- Sites like the fingers, toes, sole of the foot, and ear also need separate surgical considerations.
- 15–30% of patients with stage I and II melanoma will have some form of recurrence or metastasis during their clinical course, despite adequate surgical resection of the primary melanoma.
- Routine laboratory tests and imaging studies are not required for asymptomatic patients with primary cutaneous melanoma 4 mm or less in thickness for initial staging or routine follow-up. Indications for such studies are directed by a thorough medical history and complete physical examination.
- Elective lymph node dissection (ELND) is defined as the removal of regional lymph nodes draining the site of the primary melanoma in the absence of any clinical evidence of nodal metastases. This is a much-debated topic in the management of melanoma.

Some studies have shown increased prognosis, but other studies have shown no statistical difference.
- Sentinel lymph node biopsy (SLNB): this is based on the premise that the first node draining a lymphatic basin (sentinel lymph node) would be expected to predict the absence or presence of melanoma in that area. One per cent isosulfan blue (Lymphazurin) dye is injected around the cutaneous lesion to allow intraoperative localisation of this sentinel lymph node. Alternatively, a radioactive tracer, technetium-99, can be injected at the lesion site. A gamma probe is used to pinpoint the radiolabelled lymph node, which is then removed for histopathological review. If no melanoma cells are found, no further surgery is done. However, if the node does have involvement, the remainder of the nodes in this area are removed.
- Determination of the status of the sentinel lymph node is relevant because:
  - it has been shown to be an important independent prognostic factor, with a positive result predictive of high risk of treatment failure
  - it is a relatively low-risk procedure that can help identify high-risk patients who might benefit from additional therapy like selective complete lymphadenectomy or adjuvant interferon alpha-2b
  - it provides a psychological benefit for the patient whose sentinel lymph node biopsy does not reveal metastases.
- SLNB is viewed to be a low-yield procedure in most thin melanomas because positivity rates for sentinel lymph node biopsy are less than 5% for AJCC T1 melanomas.

### Adjuvant therapy interferon
- May improve the survival of patients with melanoma >4 mm thick.
- Diminishes the occurrence of metastases.
- Prolongs the disease-free survival in patients with melanoma >1.5 mm.

### Chemotherapy
- Advanced Stage III (unresectable regional metastases) or Stage IV (distant metastases).
- Dacarbazine remains the most active chemotherapeutic agent for the treatment of advanced melanoma. The response rate is in the range of 10% to 20%, and patients with metastases in the skin, subcutaneous tissues, or lymph nodes respond most frequently.
- Other combination chemotherapy and biochemotherapy regimens could achieve higher response rates, but do not appear to lead to durable remission.

### Biological therapy
Therapy directed toward modulating or inducing the immune system against melanoma.
- Interleukin-2 (IL-2) as a single agent has been utilised in metastatic melanoma. In one study, there was a complete response in 7% of patients, which was durable with patients remaining disease free for up to 8 years after initiating therapy.
- Another study also showed positive results by treating patients with their own tumour-infiltrating lymphocytes and IL-2.
- Monoclonal antibody therapies are, as yet, experimental and may be of potential use in melanoma.
- Melanoma vaccines have been developed to stimulate a specific response against melanoma-associated antigens. Vaccines are currently undergoing clinical trials.

### Perfusion chemotherapy
Isolated limb perfusion (ILP) has been used for melanoma of the extremities. ILP is a technique that involves isolating a limb from the systemic circulation with a tourniquet,

using arterial and venous cannulation, and infusing a chemotherapeutic agent by means of a pump oxygenator, then removing the medication from the limb. It has been developed into the most effective method of treatment for local recurrent or in-transit metastases of an extremity. Medications that are used for infusion include melphalan, dacarbazine, cisplatin, carboplatin, thiotepa, and cytokine tumour necrosis factor alpha.

**Radiation**
Radiation therapy is indicated in certain patients with stage IV disease with the purpose of palliation. Specific indications include brain metastases, pain associated with bone metastases, and skin and subcutaneous metastases that are superficially located.

# Port wine stain (naevus vinosus) and strawberry naevus

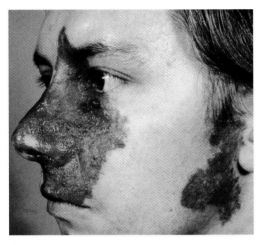

**Figure 1.11**

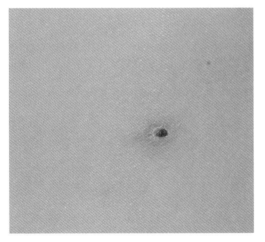

**Figure 1.12**

## Questions

**Q1** Figure 1.11 demonstrates a port wine stain. What is the abnormality?

**Q2** As the patient grows up will this lesion regress?

**Q3** Where else on the body may you find them?

**Q4** Is it associated with other congenital vascular malformations?

**Q5** Look at Figure 1.12. What is the diagnosis?

**Q6** What other types of haemangiomas are there?

## Answers

(A1) There is a capillary haemangioma just below the epidermis.

(A2) No. They tend not to regress as the patient grows up but they may fade in colour.

(A3) The junction between the limbs and trunk, lips and mucous membranes of the mouth.

(A4) Yes: Sturge–Weber syndrome is a port wine stain found in the distribution of the first and second divisions of the trigeminal nerve associated with ipsilateral intracranial haemangiomata and a history of epilepsy and/or mental retardation. It is also found on limbs in association with Klippel–Trénaunay syndrome.

(A5) Strawberry naevus: a bright red lobulated lesion that stands proud of the skin and looks like a strawberry. It is formed by a network of capillaries radiating from an artery. Present at birth, they often regress spontaneously within months or years.

(A6) 
- *Spider naevus*: a solitary dilated skin arteriole feeding a number of small branches that leave in a radial manner. It is an acquired condition associated with liver disease. In general more than five are pathological.
- *Campbell de Morgan spot*: a uniform red capillary naevus 2–3 mm in diameter. It develops on the trunk in middle age and is of no pathological significance.
- *Salmon patch*: another congenital intradermal haemangioma in which mild dilatation of the subpapillary dermal plexus gives the skin a pale pink colour. It is usually associated with other vascular abnormalities such as giant limbs, due to arteriovenous fistulae and lymphoedema.
- *Telangiectasia*: dilatation of normal capillaries. It tends to arise after irradiation. It occurs on internal mucosal surfaces as well as the skin – can lead to GI haemorrhage, haematuria and epistaxis.

# Shingles

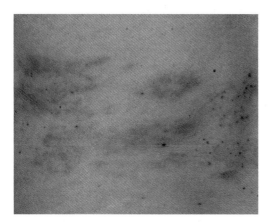

**Figure 1.13**

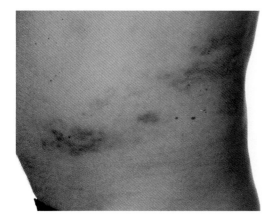

**Figure 1.14**

This 76-year-old gentleman was admitted with this rash and abdominal pain. When he stood up there was an obvious bulge to the abdominal wall.

## Questions

**Q1** What is the diagnosis?

**Q2** What are the clinical manifestations of this condition?

**Q3** What is the causative agent?

**Q4** What is the mode of transmission?

**Q5** How does it cause infection and how does each lesion progress?

## Answers

(A1) Shingles.

(A2) Initial paresis of the affected dermatome, characteristic skin eruption of a vesicular rash with vesicle scabs that usually resolve. Pain precedes the rash, is severe and sometimes persists for years as post-herpetic neuralgia.

(A3) Varicella zoster virus (VZV): this is an alpha herpes virus that infects mucous membranes, skin and neurons.

(A4) VZV is transmitted in epidemic fashion by aerosols, disseminates haematogenously and causes widespread vesicular skin lesions – chickenpox.

(A5) VZV infects satellite cells around neurons in the dorsal root ganglia and may recur many years after the primary infection in the form of shingles. Each lesion progresses rapidly from a macule to a vesicle, which resembles 'a dew drop on a rose petal'.

# Pilonidal disease

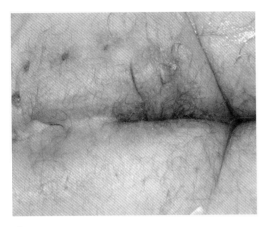

**Figure 1.15**

## Questions

(Q1) What does this photograph depict?

(Q2) How does this condition develop and where else can it occur?

(Q3) How do these patients normally present?

(Q4) This gentleman had presented 10 months earlier with an abscess in the same region. What would your management have been at the time?

(Q5) This gentleman then came to follow-up clinic with a healed scar following incision and drainage but continuing symptoms. What options would you explain are available to him?

(Q6) What is the Karydakis procedure?

(Q7) What are the other surgical options?

## Answers

 Pilonidal disease showing multiple midline pits.

 There are two schools of thought:
- *congenital*: a nest of hairs becomes enclosed as the skin closes over it. This does not explain why the hairs found at the bottom of a pilonidal abscess are demonstrably head hairs. Hence this is not the present view
- *acquired*: chronic trauma allows a hair tip to penetrate the skin and the rolling motion of the buttocks causes the hairs to burrow in. A deep natal cleft, hairy area and occupations involving prolonged sitting also predispose to this condition.

It is also found in the finger webs of people in certain occupations – hairdressers and sheepshearers, and may be also seen in the umbilicus, axilla and perianal areas.

 Patients are asymptomatic or with acute abscesses or a chronic discharging sinus.

- The immediate aim is to drain the abscess and relieve the pain by incision and drainage, with no attempt to do any more than this.
- Attempt to make the incision away from the midline.

 **Conservative**
- Minimal symptoms.
- Look for midline pits and lateral tracks. If the patient has midline pit disease and symptoms are not that bad, he can be managed conservatively with good personal hygiene and regular removal of hairs.

**Surgical**
- Usually required for ongoing symptoms.
- Lay open wound and packing, completely excising pits and lateral tracks with elliptical excision.
- Primary closure: patient should be warned of the possibility of failure as midline wounds are difficult to heal.

 The Karydakis procedure is one of several types of operation for pilonidal disease with the intent of primary closure. An advancement flap is created so that the wound is away from the midline without being under tension so that healing is improved. The natal cleft is also rendered shallow.
- Pre-operatively, the patient is given a phosphate enema to clear out the bowels to prevent early post-operative defecation.
- Intravenous antibiotic is given at induction to include anaerobic cover.
- The patient is placed prone on the table under general anaesthetic with the buttocks taped apart. The natal cleft area is depilated, prepared and draped, and any areas of infection are covered. An asymmetric ('D'-shaped) ellipse is drawn on the skin to encompass both the midline pits and lateral sinus (wider part of the ellipse). The skin is incised according to the marked pattern such that tissue is removed down to the pre-sacral fascia. The tissue beneath the flap is undermined until it can be approximated to the other side. The restraining tapes are removed, and the buttocks freed.
- Closure is with interrupted 1/0 vicryl to fat, nylon to skin. A mini-vac is placed and secured beforehand to help close down the dead space.
- The drain is reviewed and normally taken out at 24 hours.
- 5/7 of antibiotics are given.
- The patient is warned to lie on his side, with no sitting for at least 5/7 to prevent excess tension on the wound.

 Bascombe's repair and excision with advancement flaps.

# Pyoderma gangrenosum

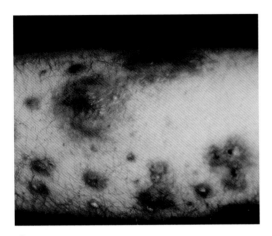

**Figure 1.16**

This patient with inflammatory bowel disease was found to have these lesions.

## Questions

**Q1** What is the lesion called and what typical points would you look for during diagnosis?

**Q2** What is the predisposing factor for its development and what other associations of the condition do you know of?

**Q3** What is the differential diagnosis?

**Q4** What other extra-intestinal manifestations of inflammatory bowel disease may occur?

**Q5** How would you treat this condition?

## Answers

**A1** Pyoderma gangrenosum

*Inspect:* ulcers with necrotic base, irregular bluish-red overhanging edges. There are normally surrounding erythematous plaques with pustules.

**A2** Immune system depression.

Associated diseases include idiopathic (50%), inflammatory bowel disease, rheumatoid arthritis, autoimmune hepatitis and myeloproliferative disorders. It is more common in males than females.

**A3**
- Autoimmune:
  - rheumatoid vasculitis.
- Infectious:
  - tertiary syphilis
  - amoebiasis.
- Iatrogenic:
  - warfarin necrosis.
- Unknown:
  - Behçet's disease.

**A4** **Manifestations related to disease activity**
- Skin: pyoderma and erythema nodosum. Mucous membranes may develop aphthous ulcers.
- Iritis.
- Arthritis of large joints.

**Manifestations unrelated to disease activity**
- Sacroiliitis.
- Ankylosing spondylitis.
- Chronic active hepatitis.
- Liver cirrhosis.
- Sclerosing cholangitis.
- Bile duct carcinoma.

Crohn's disease has an increased incidence of renal amyloidosis, and finger clubbing may occur.

**A5**
- *Medical:* treat underlying condition, saline cleansing, high-dose oral or intralesional steroids +/– cyclosporin +/– antibiotics.
- *Surgical:* serial allograft followed by autologous skin graft or muscle flap coverage when necessary.

# Erythema ab igne

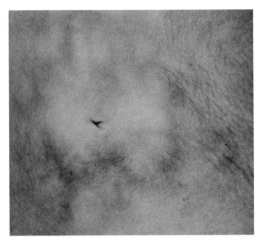

**Figure 1.17**

## Questions

**Q1** What sign does this photograph demonstrate in a patient with chronic lower abdominal pain?

**Q2** What is the explanation of the pain?

**Q3** What other signs may be present?

## Answers

**(A1)** Erythema ab igne following the application of a hot water bottle to relieve pain in the area.

**(A2)** Radiation of pain along a nerve tract that is compressed by intra-abdominal pathology.

**(A3)** The patient may have lost weight because the pain is preventing them from eating.

## Xanthelasma

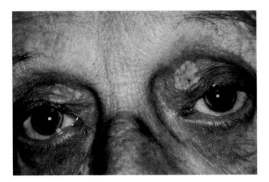

**Figure 1.18**

### Questions

Q1  What do you see in the picture?

Q2  What condition is thought to be commonly associated with xanthelasma?

Q3  What are the surgical implications in a patient who has xanthelasma?

## Answers

**(A1)** Xanthelasma palpebrarum.

**(A2)** Hyperlipoproteinaemic states, even though in the majority of patients no systemic cause can be found. Other conditions that can give rise to these include primary biliary cirrhosis.

**(A3)** Xanthelasma in a patient should alert us to underlying lipid/lipoprotein disorder. If they are seen along with other xanthomas (back of hands, buttocks, thigh and Achilles tendon) then it could suggest primary dyslipoproteinaemias. They are more prone to atherosclerotic diseases thereby increasing the risks associated with surgery.

# Lipoma

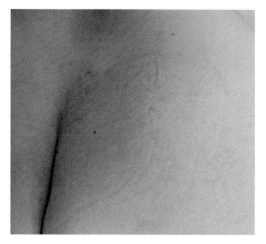

**Figure 1.19**

## Questions

**Q1** Figures 1.19 and 1.20 show the same condition. What is the diagnosis?

**Q2** What clinical findings would you expect to find?

**Q3** If this patient had multiple painful lesions what syndrome would you suspect?

**Q4** What is the probability of malignant change?

**Q5** What features might make you concerned that the lesion might be malignant?

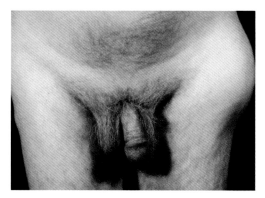

**Figure 1.20**

## Answers

(A1) A lipoma (Figure 1.19 = over right gluteal area; Figure 1.20 = over left hip area).

(A2)
- Mobile.
- Lobular.
- Soft to palpation.

(A3) Dercum's disease. This is familial.

(A4) Malignant change does not occur in lipomas.

(A5)
- Large lesion, rapidly growing, reduced mobility.
- Deep seated, particularly in lower limb tissues.
- Elderly patients.

## Umbilical hernia

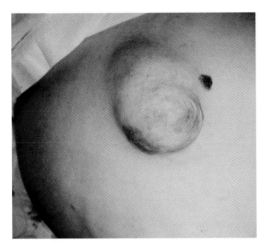

**Figure 1.21**

This patient is overweight and noticed this bulge upon coughing.

### Questions

- **Q1** What is it?
- **Q2** What is the underlying pathogenesis?
- **Q3** What does it usually contain?
- **Q4** Is this dangerous to the patient?
- **Q5** What is the condition called at this site when it occurs in children?
- **Q6** In children, is surgical intervention required in all cases?
- **Q7** What differences are there in adults?
- **Q8** How would you surgically repair it?

## Answers

**(A1)** Umbilical hernia.

**(A2)** 
- Defect through the linea alba adjacent to the umbilicus and usually due to obesity stretching the fibres.
- Uncommon before the age of 40 years.
- Can grow to an enormous size. Visible peristalsis when defect is large.

**(A3)** Nearly always omentum. In large hernias it often contains transverse colon and small bowel.

**(A4)** The neck of the sac is often narrow and held with a fibrous band. It is prone to becoming irreducible and strangulated.

**(A5)** Congenital umbilical hernia: results from failure of complete closure of the umbilical cicatrix.

**(A6)** No.
Most cases of congenital umbilical hernia close spontaneously during the first year of life and require no active treatment. They should only be repaired in symptomatic children or if it persists in a child reaching school-going age.

**(A7)** Acquired umbilical herniae may be caused by:
- pregnancy
- ascites
- ovarian cysts
- fibroids
- bowel distension.

They more commonly require surgical repair.

**(A8)** It is important to mention treating concurrent medical problems prior to surgery. Many of these patients have high anaesthetic risk because of significant co-morbidities.
- Mayo's repair (vest-over-pants).
- Incision: skin crease, transverse infra-umbilical ('smiling umbilicus incision').
- Deepen incision to rectus sheath and identify neck of sac.
- Open sac near neck and separate adhesions.
- Return protruding omentum/bowel to abdomen.
- Excise sac.
- Lower edge of rectus is sutured behind upper edge so that two flaps overlap.
- Use interrupted mattress long absorbable (preferably PDS) sutures.
- Large hernia – use of mesh.
- Laparoscopic repair can also be done.

## Inguinal and femoral herniae

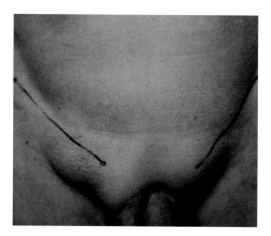

**Figure 1.22**

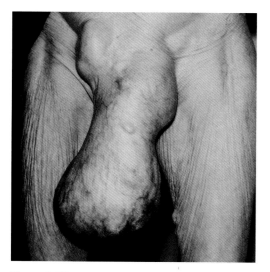

**Figure 1.23**

### Questions

**Q1** Look at Figure 1.22. What are these two swellings?

**Q2** How would you differentiate between the swellings? Which is more likely to strangulate and why?

**Q3** What are the complications of these swellings?

**Q4** What are the signs and symptoms of strangulation?

**Q5** How do you classify the swelling on the left of the patient? What are the differences?

**Q6** What are the complications of repairing the swelling on the left?

**Q7** Look at Figure 1.23. What is the diagnosis and what is the risk of strangulation?

## Answers

(A1) Right femoral hernia and left inguinal hernia.

(A2) On examination:
- *femoral hernia*: lies below and lateral to pubic tubercle
- *inguinal hernia*: lies above and medial to pubic tubercle.

Points to note:
- *inguinal hernia*: usually reducible; M:F = 6:1; risk of strangulation is low and cough impulse present
- *femoral hernia*: usually not reducible; M:F = 4:1 (but inguinal herniae are still commoner in females than femoral herniae); risk of strangulation is high and cough impulse is usually absent. Neck of hernia is usually narrower.

(A3) Intestinal obstruction and strangulation. The femoral hernia is particularly at risk because usually they have narrow necks.

(A4) Hernia is irreducible, tense and tender. Pain is severe – either colicky or can become constant. Signs suggestive of involvement of a larger segment of bowel include:
- elevation of temperature
- tachycardia
- tenderness, rigidity or rebound tenderness
- raised WCC + CRP
- shock state.

(A5) 
- Indirect.
- Direct.
- Pantaloon (combination of both).

**Indirect herniae**
- Remnants of a patent processus vaginalis.
- Arise from the abdominal cavity, passing obliquely through the deep inguinal ring *lateral* to the inferior epigastric vessels and travel through the inguinal canal with the spermatic cord.
- May continue through the supeficial ring into the scrotum.

**Direct herniae**
- Result of a weak posterior wall to the inguinal canal.
- Hernia is not within the spermatic cord but bulges through the wall into the inguinal canal *medial* to the inferior epigastric vessels.

(A6) Complications of inguinal hernia repair should be divided into immediate (first 24 hours), early (within the first month) and late (later than the first month). Furthermore there are general and specific complications of the procedure itself.

Specific complications to mention include:
- urinary retention
- bruising (30%)
- pain: acute (post-operative); chronic groin pain persists beyond 1 year in up to 5% of patients
- haematoma (10%)

- infection
- ischaemic orchitis: 0.5% – caused by thrombosis of the pampiniform plexus draining the testis
  - previous vasectomy is a predisposing cause
  - dissection beyond the pubic tubercle is one operative risk
  - more common with recurrent hernia repairs therefore should explain risk of orchidectomy
- recurrence (should be less than 0.5%)
  - normally due to inadequate deep ring and posterior wall closure
  - occasionally due to overtight sutures
- local numbness.

 Large inguino-scrotal hernia. Low risk for strangulation. This usually has a wide neck and is likely to have developed over a long period of time. Repair only if symptomatic especially in the case of the elderly. Reducing a large amount of bowel back into the abdominal cavity can cause respiratory problems

**Your revision notes:**

## Liposarcoma

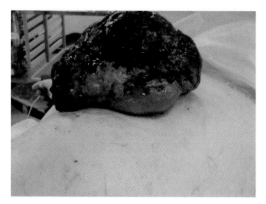

**Figure 1.24**

This patient presented with this rapidly-growing firm fixed swelling.

### Questions

(Q1) What is the most likely diagnosis?

(Q2) Name other similar type of tumours.

(Q3) Classify these tumours.

(Q4) Describe your management plan.

## Answers

 Liposarcoma of the upper thigh.
- The firm fixed nature of the swelling suggests a sarcoma. Soft tissue sarcomas are rare with an incidence of 1–3 per 100 000 population and are commonly seen in the thigh (60%). When these tumours arise from beneath the deep fascia and are fixed to the deeper structures they may be mistaken for bone tumours.
- They are more common in males with a ratio of 2:1 and a predilection to older patients.

- Malignant histiocytoma: commonest.
- Synovial sarcoma.
- Fibrosarcoma: malignant tumours of the fibrous tissue. The high-grade fibrosarcomas have poorer prognosis. Excision with clear margins is the treatment. However recurrence is as high as 46%.
- Rhabdomyosarcoma: it is a malignant tumour of the muscle. It is commoner in the thigh, shoulder and the upper arm. MRI may be helpful. Treatment is surgical but it has poor prognosis.

 They are histologically classified into:
- well differentiated
- myxoid
- round cell
- pleomorphic.

The well-differentiated tumours are composed of mature adipocytes and have a good prognosis. They do not metastasise and grow locally. The second subtype, myxoid variety, is composed of pleomorphic adipocytes and fibroblast-like cells. They may metastasise.

The pleomorphic liposarcoma is the least differentiated and the most malignant type. Mortality is 77% in this subtype.

These tumours commonly occur in the lower extremities and also in the retroperitoneum. These tumours usually metastasise via the haematogenous route and the commonest site is the lung.

 **Investigations**
- Histopathological study of biopsy sample: the purpose of the biopsy is to obtain enough tissue to determine the histological type and grade of the lesion.
- MRI may be helpful in planning treatment since it may demonstrate spread along tissue planes.
- Staging CT for distant metastasis: the staging system used is the AJC/UICC (American Joint Committee/Union Internationale Contre le Cancer) and is based on histological grade (G), size of the tumour (T), involvement of the regional nodes and also distant metastasis.

**Treatment**
- Treatment of the primary tumour is by wide excision. This gives the best chance of a cure. This will usually require some sort of plastic reconstruction to restore skin cover over the area.
- For the treatment of less differentiated tumours, radiotherapy may be considered along with surgery.
- Chemotherapy is as yet of little proven value, however it has been used more commonly recently.

# Neurofibromatosis

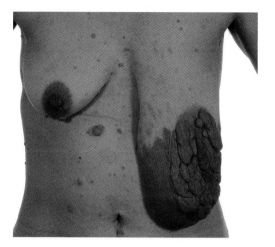

**Figure 1.25**

## Questions

**Q1** What is the diagnosis?

**Q2** What is the underlying problem? What are the different types?

**Q3** What complications can a patient with this problem develop?

**Q4** How would you treat a patient with a single lesion?

**Q5** What are the important associations of this condition?

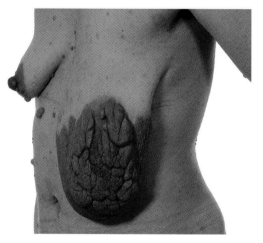

**Figure 1.26**

## Answers

 Neurofibromatosis.

 This is the presence of multiple neurofibromas in a patient in combination with other dermatological manifestations (six café-au-lait spots). It is an autosomal dominant condition. There are two types:
- *type I:* (von Recklinghausen's disease): defective gene on chromosome 17
- *type II:* defective gene on chromosome 22 with variable penetrance – fewer cutaneous signs seen.

A neurofibroma is a benign tumour derived from peripheral nerve elements.

 • Pressure effects: spinal cord or nerve root compression.
- Deafness with involvement of VIIIth cranial nerve.
- Sarcomatous transformation: only in type I disease (5–15%).
- Intra-abdominal effects: obstruction, chronic gastrointestinal bleeds.
- Skeletal changes: kyphoscoliosis, cystic changes and pseudoarthrosis.

 • Non-surgical: if asymptomatic and patient wishes to leave alone.
- Surgical: indicated if malignant growth is suspected. Malignant degeneration may occur in up to 10%. However after excision, regrowth is common as neurofibromata cannot be detached from the underlying nerve.

 • Association with medullary carcinoma of the thyroid/phaeochromocytoma as part of MEN Type IIb syndrome.
- Higher incidence of gliomas and meningiomas in patients with neurofibromas.

## Clubbing

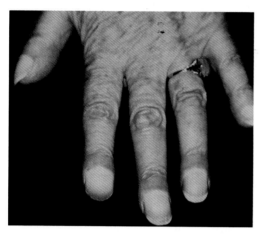

Figure 1.27

### Questions

Q1  What is the clinical sign being demonstrated?

Q2  Describe the changes you see in this condition during observation and on palpation.

Q3  What else would you like to examine?

Q4  What are the possible causes?

Q5  What do you know about the underlying pathophysiology of this condition?

## Answers

 Digital clubbing: the word 'clubbing' on its own may have several connotations, e.g. something done on a Friday night!

- Exaggerated antero-posterior and longitudinal curvature to the fingernails.
- Loss of angle between the nail and nail bed.
- Drumstick or parrot beak appearance of the nail (aka doigts Hippocratique).
- On palpation: increased bogginess/fluctuation of nail bed.

- Palpate wrist joints for tenderness in HPOA: rapid painful digital clubbing is nearly always due to bronchial carcinoma.
- Examine toes for digital clubbing.
- History and examination to look for duration (?since birth) and for underlying causes.

- *Cardiovascular*: congenital cyanotic heart disease, infective endocarditis, atrial myxoma (rare).
- *Respiratory*: fibrosing alveolitis, chronic suppurative lung disease, e.g. bronchiectasis, bronchial carcinoma (most commonly squamous cell), pleural and mediastinal tumours.
- *Gastrointestinal*: liver cirrhosis (especially primary biliary cirrhosis), liver failure, inflammatory bowel disease (Crohn's disease), gastrointestinal lymphoma, malabsorption (coeliac disease, tropical sprue).
- *Idiopathic*: most common cause!
- *Congenital*.

**Rarer causes**
- *Familial*: 'hazel nails' usually seen before puberty.
- *Pachydermoperiostitis*: idiopathic familial HPOA with post-pubertal digital clubbing, bone changes, increased sweating of palms and soles, and marked thickening of the skin, forehead and scalp.
- *Graves' disease*: pseudoclubbing – thyroid acropachy.
- Unilaterally seen in axillary artery aneurysm and brachial arteriovenous malformation.

 Several theories have been put forward to explain the mechanism behind digital clubbing:
- vasodilatation of nail bed vessels secondary to an unidentified mediator ?bradykinin, prostaglandin, 5-HT. Normally inactivated in lung but may persist in those with clubbing where inactivation is defective or where there is a right to left shunt
- increased growth hormone
- tumour necrosis factor
- increased platelet-derived growth factor and FGF resulting in increased fibroblastic activity, capillary permeability and arterial smooth muscle hyperplasia
- organs supplied by the vagus nerve are affected by digital clubbing – vagotomy can reverse digital clubbing in bronchial carcinoma.

# Sebaceous cysts

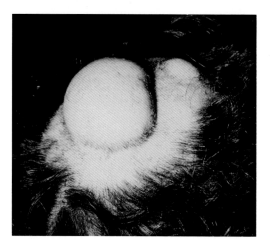

**Figure 1.28**

This woman presented with this mobile smooth hemispherical swelling on her scalp.

## Questions

Q1  What is the diagnosis?

Q2  Where else are they commonly found? Where on the skin do they never occur?

Q3  What do they look like when cut open?

Q4  What are the complications of this?

Q5  What are the different histological subtypes of this condition?

Q6  What is the name given to them when they form a fungating polypoidal mass?

Q7  How would you treat this mobile mass?

Q8  What would you do if this mass were infected?

## Answers

**(A1)** Sebaceous cyst.

**(A2)** Face, trunk, neck, scrotum and vulva. They are never found on the palms and soles.

**(A3)** There is a white lining of squamous epithelium. Contains cheese-like material and smells unpleasant.

**(A4)**
- Infection: frequent – associated with pus discharge, usually through the punctum.
- Ulceration.
- Calcification.
- Sebaceous horn formation.
- Malignant change (very rare).

**(A5)**
- *Epidermal cysts*: thought to arise from the infundibular portions of hair follicles.
- *Trichilemmal cysts*: thought to arise from hair follicle epithelium, therefore more common on the scalp. Frequently multiple. There is an autosomal dominant mode of inheritance.

**(A6)** Cock's peculiar tumour: clinically and histologically looks like a squamous cell carcinoma. Malignant transformation is very rare.

**(A7)**
- *Non-surgical*: if small and asymptomatic. However need to warn patient of risk of infection and they should consider having it removed.
- *Surgical*: usually under LA, via an elliptical incision containing the punctum. Complete excision of cyst and it contents is required to prevent recurrence.

**(A8)**
- Incision and drainage.
- Curettage of cyst wall.
- Leave wound open and pack.

# Keratoacanthoma

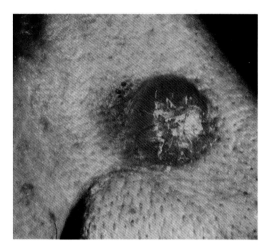

**Figure 1.29**

A 30-year-old male noticed this fast-growing non-tender lump on the right alar of his nose over the last six weeks.

## Questions

Q1 What is the most likely diagnosis?

Q2 How do you define this lesion?

Q3 What is the typical mode of presentation?

Q4 What is the cause?

Q5 What is your differential diagnosis?

Q6 How would you treat this lesion in this patient?

## Answers

(A1) A keratoacanthoma.

(A2) A benign overgrowth of hair follicle cells producing a central plug of keratin.

(A3) Usually occurs on the face but can occur anywhere where there are sebaceous glands (also known as adenoma sebaceum). The central core is hard and usually separates. The lump collapses down leaving a deep indrawn scar. It is rapidly growing; forms within six weeks and regresses spontaneously over 2–3 months. More common in males and normally single lesions.

(A4) Cause unknown. May be a self-limiting neoplasm or an unusual response to infection.

(A5) • Basal cell carcinoma: sometimes difficult to distinguish – history will help.
• Squamous cell carcinoma: grows more slowly; does not have a dead central core; gradually becomes an ulcer.

(A6) • Non-surgically: in a young patient if it is asymptomatic.
• Surgically excise lesion for histology especially in older patients when there is a higher index of suspicion for malignancy.
• Surgical excision will also result in better cosmesis.

# Femoral hernia

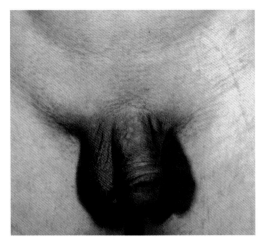

**Figure 1.30**

## Questions

**Q1** What is the diagnosis and why is this unusual in this person?

**Q2** What is the aetiology of this condition?

**Q3** Describe the boundaries of the swelling.

**Q4** What are the surgical principles and options of repairing this swelling?

**Q5** What are the complications specific to surgery for this condition?

A 45-year-old male presented to A&E with this lump in his right groin, which was irreducible and had no cough impulse. On examination it was found to be below and lateral to the pubic tubercle.

## Answers

**(A1)** The diagnosis is a femoral hernia. After inguinal hernia this is the second most common type of hernia, with a female to male predominance of 4:1. The pelvis is wider in the female than the male, therefore the femoral canal is correspondingly larger.

**(A2)** The underlying cause is a weakness of the femoral ring secondary to atrophy or dilatation. With time the transversalis fascia is forced into the canal and may be followed by peritoneum and extraperitoneal fat. This gives the characteristic thick-walled feel of the hernia.

**(A3)** This is a question related to the femoral canal – this is where a femoral hernia may arise. The boundaries are mainly ligamentous except laterally – the femoral vein. The ligamentous boundaries make strangulation more common.
- Medially: sharp edge of the lacunar part of the inguinal ligament.
- Laterally: femoral vein.
- Posteriorly: the pectineal ligament of Astley Cooper.
- Anteriorly: inguinal ligament.

**(A4)** Surgical principles of femoral hernia repair are:
1 reduction of the contents of the sac
2 excision of the sac
3 repair of defect: taking care not to narrow the femoral vein while tightening up the femoral canal.

**Surgical approaches**
- *Crural or low approach*: incision made directly over the hernia. Easiest approach and best option for elective procedures but risk of narrowing the femoral vein when closing the femoral canal.
- *Abdominal or pre-peritoneal repair* (McEvedy): best technique for strangulated herniae as it can be converted to a more extensive operation seeking any ischaemic bowel by making a second incision.
- *Inguinal or high approach*: posterior wall of the inguinal canal is opened to access the femoral canal from above. Best approach if the nature of the hernia is uncertain as inguinal hernia can also be repaired. Recurrent inguinal herniae are common.

**(A5)**
- Damage to an accessory obturator artery if present.
- Bladder perforation.
- Femoral vein injury or stenosis.

## Pyogenic granuloma

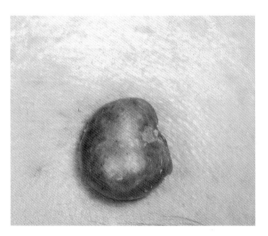

**Figure 1.31**

### Questions

**Q1** What is the most likely diagnosis?

**Q2** Where are these lesions commonly found?

**Q3** What are the pertinent points on clinical examination?

**Q4** What questions would you ask the patient?

**Q5** How would you treat this condition?

This photograph is from a nine-year-old boy who attended outpatients with this bright red lesion on his face which had appeared over the preceding three weeks.

## Answers

(A1) Pyogenic granuloma: this is a rapidly growing capillary haemangioma which usually measures less than 1 cm in diameter.

(A2)
- Hands and face in children and young adults.
- Gums and lips in pregnant women.

(A3) **Inspection**
- Bright red hemispherical nodule.
- Sessile or pedunculated.
- May be associated with a serous or purulent discharge.
- Can epithelialise if long-standing (skin colour).

**Palpation**
- Soft consistency.
- Compressible: due to vascular origin.
- May bleed!

(A4) Ask:
- previous injury to area? – link to trauma
- how long did the lump take to appear? – rapid growth in a few days
- how lump affects patient's life – pain, cosmesis, bleeding?

(A5)
- *Non-surgical*: silver nitrate stick.
- *Surgical*:
  - regression is uncommon except in pregnancy; best treated surgically
  - curettage with diathermy to base
  - complete excision biopsy.

If recurrent need to consider malignancy – amelanotic melanoma.

## Rectus sheath haematoma

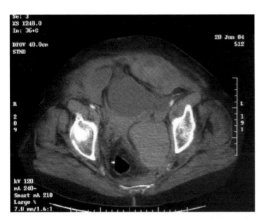

**Figure 1.32**

### Questions

**Q1** What is the diagnosis?

**Q2** What are the clinical features?

**Q3** How do you investigate this condition?

**Q4** What are the treatment options?

A 72-year-old lady presented with sudden onset of lower abdominal pain after a bout of coughing. Abdominal pain was associated with extensive bruising and fullness in the lower abdomen. The patient has been on warfarin for atrial fibrillation. A CT of the abdomen was performed.

## Answers

 Bilateral rectus sheath haematoma: it is an uncommon, but not rare, cause of abdominal pain.

 **Symptoms**
- Fever and chills are common.
- History of straining or paroxysm of coughing.
- Severe lower abdominal pain associated with bruising. The pain is severe with an associated palpable mass.
- Anorexia, nausea, vomiting, diarrhoea, constipation are all compatible with the diagnosis of this condition.

**Signs**
- A low-grade fever is common.
- If the haematoma is large there may be signs of hypovolumic shock including hypotension and tachycardia.
- Abdominal examination reveals a palpable, painful mass corresponding to the rectus sheath. A tender swelling develops usually below the umbilicus (the swelling is usually posterior to the muscle and hence difficult to palpate). Rarely the haematoma can rupture and cause signs of peritonitis.
- Fothergill's sign is elicited by having the patient raise the head while in a supine position. Intra-abdominal masses will become impalpable and abdominal wall masses will be fixed and palpable. A tender mass that does not disappear with contraction of the rectus muscles is indicative of a rectus sheath haematoma.
- It usually develops from a rupture of the branches of the superior or inferior epigastric artery.
- They can be spontaneous (haemophiliacs, leukaemics, in patients on anticoagulants), after mild straining such as coughing, direct violence or, rarely, direct tear of rectus muscle.
- It is 2–3 times more common in females. Pregnancy is a risk factor, however in males it is more common after trauma or muscular exertion. Peak incidence is in the 5th decade of life.

- Haematology:
  - FBC
  - coagulation profile.
- Imaging:
  - ultrasonography: the first line investigation and can help in establishing the diagnosis
  - CT scanning: better than ultrasound as it gives the location, extent and size of the haematoma. It is 100% sensitive and 100% specific in acute rectus sheath haematoma
  - MRI is useful in differentiating chronic haematomas from other abdominal wall conditions.

 Once rectus sheath haematoma is diagnosed, the patient's clinical condition dictates further management. Treatment may be conservative or invasive.

**Conservative**
In patients who are haemodynamically stable:
- ice packs
- control of pain
- resuscitation

- reversal of anticoagulation
- transfusion.

The haematomas usually settle in 3–4 weeks.

**Invasive**
In patients who are unstable and also if the haematoma is expanding (due to active bleeding):
- gelfoam embolisation of the bleeding vessel
- operative exploration: evacuation of haematoma, ligation of bleeding vessels.

This condition is usually a benign self-limiting condition. The increase in morbidity is due to incorrect diagnosis. The mortality rates have decreased since the advent of ultrasonography and CT for imaging.

**Your revision notes:**

# Ganglion

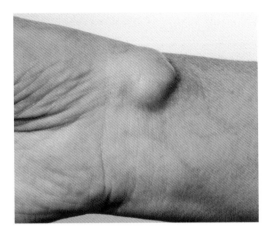

**Figure 1.33**

A 45-year-old gentleman presented with this swelling over his right wrist.

## Questions

(Q1) What is the diagnosis?

(Q2) What is the differential diagnosis?

(Q3) How do these lesions typically present?

(Q4) What is the origin of this swelling?

(Q5) Where else are they seen on the body?

(Q6) How would you treat this condition?

(Q7) What complications are associated with surgical treatment?

## Answers

(A1) A ganglion.

(A2) • Bursae.
• Cystic protrusions from the synovial cavity of arthritic joints.
• Benign giant cell tumours of the flexor sheath.
• Rare malignant swellings, e.g. synovial sarcoma.
• Beware of a rare radial artery aneurysm!

(A3) Young adult presenting with a tense painless swelling on the dorsum of wrist.

(A4) A ganglion is a cystic swelling related to a synovial lined cavity – either a joint or a tendon sheath. The origin is controversial: benign tumour of the joint capsule or tendon sheath or a degenerative process of the tendon sheath/joint capsule secondary to trauma.

(A5) Other common sites include dorsum of foot, flexor aspect of the fingers and over the peroneal tendons.

(A6) **Non-surgical**
• Watchful waiting policy if the ganglion does not affect patient's life.
• Aspiration followed by three weeks of immobilisation (30–50% successful).

**Surgical**
• Complete excision to include the neck of the ganglion at its site of origin under local anaesthetic.

(A7) • Wound complications: scar, haematoma, infection.
• Recurrence: can be as high as 1/3 if not excised completely.

## Hidradenitis suppurativa

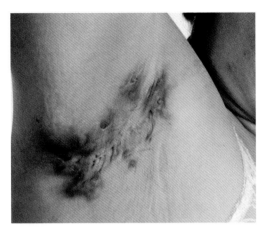

**Figure 1.34**

### Questions

(Q1) What is the diagnosis?

(Q2) What is the underlying aetiology?

(Q3) What are the predisposing factors of this condition?

(Q4) What other regions of the body does this condition commonly affect?

(Q5) What are the treatment options?

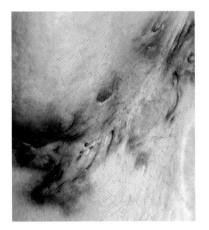

**Figure 1.35**

## Answers

(A1)   Hidradenitis suppurativa.

(A2)   • This is a chronic and recurrent infection of the apocrine sweat glands. It is thought to be due to an antigen–antibody reaction with subsequent blockage of follicular secretions and subsequent abscess formation.
   • Repeated infection creates a wide area of inflamed and scarred tissue which is foul-smelling and painful.
   • Other theories are based on the concept that it is due to a defect of terminal follicular epithelium.

(A3)   • HS is not seen before puberty and most patients are aged 16–40 years.
   • Usually affects young women. Prevalence of 0.5% in industrialised countries.
   • Obesity, acne, poor hygiene, excessive sweating, diabetes mellitus have been suggested as pre-disposing factors.

(A4)   • Axilla most common site.
   • Other sites that can be affected are the groin, perineum, back of neck and umbilicus.

(A5)   HS can be very difficult to treat:
   • for well-localised abscess: incision and drainage under antibiotic cover
   • larger lesions: radical excision with either primary closure or full-thickness skin grafting usually harvested from groin or abdomen
   • despite radical surgery there is a significant recurrence rate depending on site affected:
      – inguinal and perineal regions: up to 50%
      – lowest for axillary region.

## Keloid and hypertrophic scars

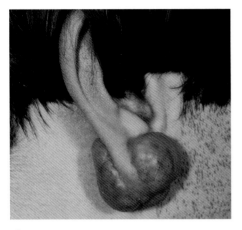

**Figure 1.36**

### Questions

**Q1** Look at Figures 1.36 and 1.37. What are the diagnoses?

**Q2** What are the distinguishing features between the two?

**Q3** Is there a difference in the clinical course between the two?

**Q4** What are the predisposing factors?

**Q5** How do you treat this problem?

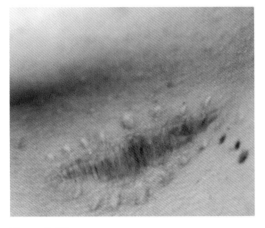

**Figure 1.37**

## Answers

**A1**
- Figure 1.36: keloid scar over right earlobe.
- Figure 1.37: hypertrophic scar.

**A2**
- *Hypertrophic scar*: scar confined to wound margins and normally found across flexor surfaces and skin creases.
- *Keloid scar*: scar extends beyond wound margins and normally located on ear lobes, chin, neck, shoulder and chest, anterior abdominal wall – commonly in the midline.

**A3** Hypertrophic scars normally appear soon after injury and usually regress spontaneously, while keloid scars have the tendency to appear months after injury and are likely to grow further.

**A4** Wounds associated with:
- tension, e.g. sternotomy wounds after cardiothoracic surgery. Thought to be due to relative tissue hypoxia
- burns
- trauma
- infection
- wounds on certain sites of the body (see A2)
- post-radiotherapy
- post-BCG inoculation.

Other associations include:
- genetic: keloid scars more common in Black and Hispanic races
- children
- pregnancy
- immunological: increase in IgG, IgM, ANA and C3 levels to keloid fibroblasts.

**A5** Recurrence rate after surgery alone can be up to 55%, therefore combination therapy is often employed.

### Non-surgical
- Mechanical pressure therapy, topical silicone gel sheets.
- Intralesional steroid and local anaesthetic injections using triamcinolone in combination with lidocaine.

### Surgical
- Scar revision with primary closure of scar, local Z-plasty or skin grafting to avoid excessive tension.

# Section 2

# Upper GI tract and hepatobiliary system

# Sengstaken–Blakemore tube

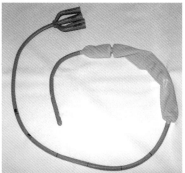

**Figure 2.1**

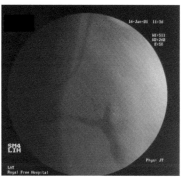

**Figure 2.5**

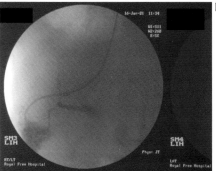

**Figure 2.2**

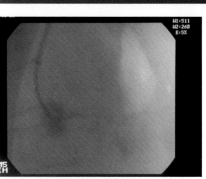

**Figure 2.3**

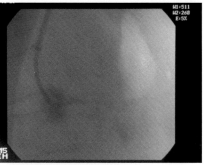

**Figure 2.4**

## Questions

**Q1** Identify the object shown in Figure 2.1.

**Q2** What are its clinical uses?

**Q3** How does it control haemorrhage in these cases? Can it be left inflated indefinitely?

**Q4** What is the purpose of the narrow distal end of the tube, which leads into the stomach?

**Q5** How else can this source of haematemesis be dealt with?

**Q6** What radiological procedure is depicted in Figures 2.2 to 2.5? Are there any disadvantages to this procedure?

**Q7** What is the outlook following a variceal bleed?

**Q8** Should patients with oesophageal varices that have not bled be treated?

## Answers

(A1) A Sengstaken–Blakemore tube.

(A2) In patients with haematemesis due to bleeding oesophageal and gastric varices in portal hypertension.

(A3) It causes a mechanical tamponade. It consists of a nasogastric tube with two large balloons at the distal end. Two balloons – one in the oesophagus and one in the cardia – are blown up to compress the varices. The tube position must be confirmed by radiograph before inflation of the balloons. The distal gastric balloon is inflated with 250 ml of air and then pulled up tight against the gastro-oesophageal junction. If the gastric balloon alone does not control the bleeding, the proximal oesophageal balloon is inflated to a pressure that equals portal venous pressure (25 mmHg). The tube is deflated at 24 hours, and if bleeding has stopped it is removed 48 hours after insertion. If bleeding is not controlled, the tube is left inflated for a further 24 hours after an interval of 1 hour deflation. It cannot be left inflated indefinitely – complications of balloon tamponade are ischaemic necrosis of the oesophageal mucosa, oesophageal perforation and aspiration pneumonitis.

(A4) It is a gastric tube that is used to aspirate the stomach or for feeding purposes.

(A5)
- Use of a fibreoptic oesophagoscope and injection of sclerosant (injection sclerotherapy) or variceal banding.
- Drug treatments: aim to reduce variceal blood pressure and flow; somatostatin and its analogues such as octreotide. Vasopressin has been used to reduce portal pressure.
- Emergency operations are a last resort in variceal bleed and are rarely performed these days. Procedures performed include lower oesophageal transection or an emergency portosystemic shunting procedure.

(A6)
- Transjugular intrahepatic porto-systemic shunting (TIPSS). This is an alternative to surgical shunting. This shunts portal blood across the liver into the vena cava.
- A guide wire introduced through the jugular vein is threaded through the liver and forced into an intrahepatic branch of the portal vein. This track is balloon dilated and held open with a metallic stent, creating a shunt that decompresses the portal system. Use with caution – can worsen an encephalopathy. Also only a temporary measure – shunts thrombose within 1 year.

(A7) Mortality from a first variceal bleed is around 50%. Those that survive have an overall 70% risk of further bleeding and so should be aggressively treated. Repeated endoscopic sclerotherapy or banding of varices should be undertaken until all visible vessels are eradicated. Prophylactic atenolol or propranolol should be given, as these have been shown both to reduce mortality from the initial bleed and reduce the risk of rebleeding. Aim also to improve the underlying portal hypertension – hepatic transplantation may be needed to achieve this.

(A8) Prophylactic shunt surgery aimed at preventing first variceal bleed results in a greater chance of dying than doing nothing. Prophylactic endoscopic sclerotherapy results in either no benefit or a deleterious effect compared with no treatment. Endoscopic band ligation prophylaxis has reduced bleeding and reduced mortality in some studies but further confirmation is required. Prophylactic treatment with β-blockers reduces the risk of a first variceal bleed and appears to improve survival. Patients with large varices are more likely to experience a first variceal bleed and therefore should be considered for preventative therapy.

## Oesophageal carcinoma

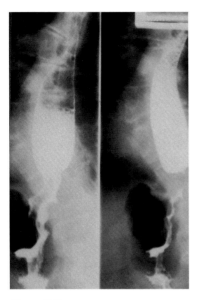

**Figure 2.6**

This investigation was performed on a 60-year-old patient with worsening dysphagia and weight loss.

### Questions

**Q1** What investigation has been performed? What does it show and what is the most likely diagnosis?

**Q2** What is the epidemiology of this condition?

**Q3** What are the risk factors for developing this condition?

**Q4** What options are available for *palliative* treatment?

**Q5** What are the indications against curative resection?

**Q6** What operations may be performed for curative resection of this disease?

**Q7** What are the most common complications following oesophagectomy?

## Answers

**A1** A barium swallow. There is hold up of contrast at the distal oesophagus with irregular narrowing of the gastro-oesophageal junction area. This needs further evaluation by an OGD and most probably represents an oesophageal carcinoma.

**A2**
- China/Iran and Caspian region 100/100 000 compared to Western Europe 5/100 000.
- M:F = 5:1 between 50 and 70 years of age.
- US black males 3× compared to white males.

**A3**
- Smoking, high alcohol intake, nitrosamines in diet, achalasia, Barrett's oesophagus, Plummer–Vinson syndrome, corrosive strictures.
- Tobacco + alcohol synergistic factors.

**A4**
- Palliative resection, bypassed with stomach (Kirschner's operation), laser therapy, oesophageal covered stent.
- External beam radiotherapy.

**A5**
- Evidence of distant metastases, e.g. supraclavicular lymph nodes.
- Co-morbidities such as severe COPD, MI in last 6 months, uncontrolled angina, a predicted LVEF <40%, hepatic cirrhosis and chronic renal failure.
- Age >75 years is also considered to be a relative contraindication for oesophagectomy.

**A6**
- Ivor–Lewis procedure: right 5th ICS thoracotomy and upper midline laparotomy (for mid- and lower-third tumours).
- Left thoraco-abdominal approach: for lower-third and cardia tumours (McEwen's procedure).
- Transhiatal approach: upper midline laparotomy and cervical incision. This avoids a thoracotomy (Orringer's procedure).

**A7**
- Bleeding.
- Respiratory problems (50%): penumothorax, pleural effusion, pneumonia.
- Anastomotic leak (5%) associated with high mortality.
- Atrial fibrillation.
- Development of an anastomotic stricture.
- Thoracic duct injury.
- Post-operative mortality in 5–10% region.
- 5-year survival following surgery around 20%.

# Gastric volvulus

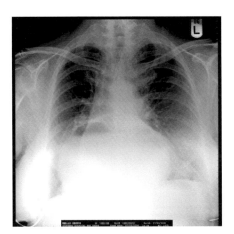

Figure 2.7

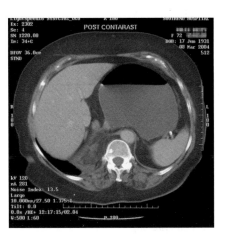

Figure 2.9

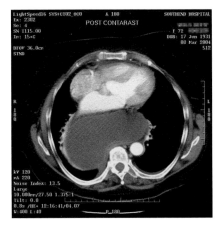

Figure 2.8

A 72-year-old female presented with sudden on-set of severe epigastric and left upper quadrant pain. The pain was sharp and constant, relieved only upon vomiting. The vomitus was projectile and streaked with blood. The only significant past medical history was of a hiatus hernia for which the patient was taking a proton pump inhibitor.

It was noted that a nasogastric tube was difficult to pass. This patient had the following chest radiograph and subsequent CT scan.

## Questions

**Q1** Describe the radiological findings (Figures 2.7–2.9).

**Q2** What is the most likely diagnosis?

**Q3** What are the incidence, classification, presentation and prognosis of this condition?

**Q4** What are the investigations of choice in this condition?

**Q5** What is the treatment of this condition?

## Answers

 • Figure 2.7: CXR – large air-fluid level behind the heart in keeping with an incarcerated hiatus hernia.
• Figure 2.8: CT-dilated stomach with fluid in it behind heart above diaphragm.
• Figure 2.9: CT-dilated gastric antrum below diaphragm.

 Strangulated gastric volvulus.

 Gastric volvulus is an uncommon surgical emergency that is potentially fatal. Diagnosis is often difficult and delayed and treatment is controversial. It occurs predominantly in older adults with other co-morbidities, which accounts for a high mortality rate of 30–50%. The stomach is abnormally rotated either along its longitudinal or transverse axis. When the rotation exceeds 180%, gastric obstruction or strangulation may occur. Strangulation is the major cause of death, leading to necrosis, perforation and hypovolaemic shock.

### Classification
• Acute or chronic.
• Primary (30%) or secondary (70%).

### Secondary causes
• Paraoesophageal hiatus hernia, traumatic diaphragmatic hernia, eventration of the diaphragm, abdominal bands or adhesions.

### Predisposing factors
• Abnormalities of the stomach: includes conditions that produce acute or chronic distension. Pyloric stenosis and duodenal obstruction produce elongation of the ligaments attached to the stomach and gastric ptosis.
• Abnormalities of the surrounding viscera, e.g. splenomegaly producing elongation of the gastrosplenic ligament.
• Rotation of the stomach to fill an abnormal space:
  – in association with a paraoesophageal hiatus hernia
  – with other forms of hiatus or diaphragmatic herniae
  – congenital or acquired eventration of the diaphragm.

### Presentation
• Acute volvulus: triad of epigastric pain, vomiting followed by retching without the ability to vomit and difficulty in passing a nasogastric tube.
• Chronic volvulus: dysphagia, vomiting, waterbrash, gastro-oesophageal reflux and breathlessness.

 The diagnosis of gastric volvulus can be difficult. Investigations of choice include plain chest radiograph, barium contrast studies, endoscopy, and computed tomography. Barium studies are thought to provide the greatest yield, whereas plain chest radiographs are more suggestive of the condition rather than being diagnostic.

 Treatment options in acute volvulus:
• Conservative.
• Surgical:
  – open
  – laparoscopic
  – combined open/laparoscopic
  – endoscopic.

- Open technique includes laparotomy for reduction of the volvulus and correction of the underlying cause, e.g. diaphragmatic hernia repair, division of bands with or without fixation of the stomach by gastropexy. In strangulation a total or partial gastrectomy may be required. There may be a concurrent need for Nissen fundoplication to treat gastro-oesophageal reflux disease (GORD), which may be a problem in patients with an underlying hiatus hernia as well as reducing the risk of recurrence.
- Gastropexy alone via PEG or laparoscopically.
- Endoscopy for reduction of the volvulus.
- Combined open and laparoscopic techniques.

In recent years less invasive techniques have been used in view of the magnitude of the surgical insult in a predominantly elderly population.

**Your revision notes:**

## Barrett's oesophagus

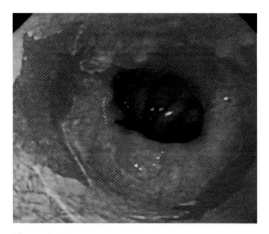

**Figure 2.10**

This photograph was taken at the time of an upper GI endoscopy of a fit 50-year-old gentleman who had been complaining of worsening reflux symptoms over the past year.

## Questions

**Q1** What does it show?

**Q2** What is the most likely diagnosis? What is the significance of this?

**Q3** What is the underlying pathogenesis of this condition? What normally prevents this condition from occurring?

**Q4** How would you manage this patient?

**Q5** What is the Savary–Miller grading system?

## Answers

 There are islands of mucosa, which look redder and more erythematous than the surrounding mucosa above the gastro-oesophageal junction.

 Barrett's oesophagus.
- This is a pre-malignant condition. The relative risk of developing adenocarcinoma of the oesophagus in patients with Barrett's is 50–100×.

- The normal surface epithelium of the oesophagus is mainly stratified squamous epithelium. This becomes columnar lined at the level of the gastro-oesophageal junction. If it occurs more than 3 cm from the junction this is thought to be abnormal and is called a classical Barrett's oesophagus.
- It is thought to occur by metaplasia (transformation of one differentiated cell type into another). The stimulus is thought to be gastro-oesophageal reflux.
- Shorter segments of metaplasia are also currently considered to be significant.
- There is a natural area of high pressure at the lower end of the oesophagus that acts as a physiological sphincter to prevent reflux of gastric contents.

- Barrett's patients should receive permanent proton pump inhibitor therapy.
- Treatment of Barrett's is controversial: few surgeons would advocate oesophagectomy for early dysplastic change. The difference between high-grade dysplasia and cancer is sometimes difficult, and severe dysplasia would warrant consideration of surgery in the setting of an MDT meeting. Most surgeons would advocate regular endoscopic surveillance once these changes have been identified. If the patient was frail and elderly and would not be fit enough to undergo oesophagectomy, repeat endoscopy is not warranted.
- Endoscopic methods to ablate the affected mucosa have also been tried.
- This patient should undergo endoscopic surveillance if the length of Barrett's is more than 3 cm, if there is intestinal metaplasia on histology, the patient is fit for surgery and understands the need for surveillance and surgery if dysplasia is found.
- Surveillance endoscopy: biopsy suspicious areas and also take quadrantic biopsies every 2 cm from the tip of the gastric folds to the squamous columnar junction.
- Follow-up depends on histology (based on BSG guidelines):
  - *no dysplasia*: 3-yearly OGD. Discharge from surveillance if co-morbidity or age rules out surgery
  - *low-grade dysplasia*: treat with PPI to reduce inflammation and repeat OGD at 6 months with quadrantic biopsies every 2 cm
  - *high-grade dysplasia*: discuss at upper GI cancer MDT meeting for collective decision.

 Used to grade endoscopic changes in GORD:
*Grade I*: erythema at the squamous–columnar junction.
*Grade II*: non-confluent linear ulceration in the lower 5 cm of the oesophagus.
*Grade III*: confluent linear ulceration in the lower 5 cm of the oesophagus.
*Grade IV*: circumferential fibrosis, stricture, Barrett's oesophagus.

## Gallstone ileus

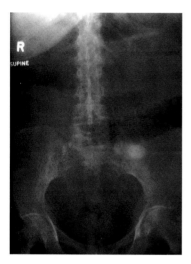

**Figure 2.11**

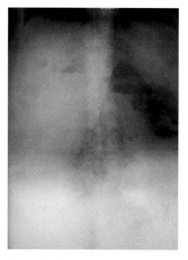

**Figure 2.12**

This 43-year-old lady presented with abdominal pain and vomiting.

## Questions

**Q1** What do these abdominal X-rays show? What is the most likely diagnosis?

**Q2** What proportion of cases of small bowel obstruction has this aetiology?

**Q3** What are the other possible causes for the main finding on the film?

**Q4** What are the pathological changes responsible for bringing about this condition?

**Q5** How would you treat this patient?

## Answers

(A1)
- Air in the biliary tree.
- Calcifications in the abdomen suspicious for gallstones.
- Small bowel obstruction with air-fluid levels.

Appearances are suspicious for gallstone ileus.

(A2) 1%.

(A3)
- Ascending cholangitis.
- Biliary-intestinal bypass.
- ERCP with sphincterotomy.

(A4) Gallstone fistulates into the small bowel (duodenum) directly, it does not pass through the biliary tree. The gallstone lodges in the terminal ileum causing obstruction.

(A5)
- Laparotomy and enterotomy proximal to the site of impaction. Milk the gallstone proximally. Then close the enterotomy.
- Do not perform cholecystectomy at this point because it is technically very difficult and probably unnecessary as a fistula has already formed.

## Chronic pancreatitis

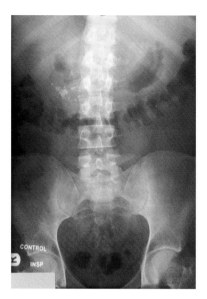

**Figure 2.13**

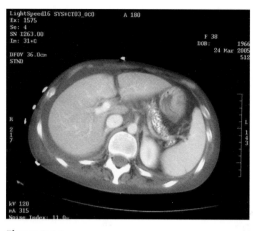

**Figure 2.14**

This 32-year-old lady attended outpatients with an epigastric mass. Radiology is shown in Figures 2.13 and 2.14.

## Questions

**Q1** What does the imaging show? What is the most likely diagnosis?

**Q2** What is the most common cause of this condition?

**Q3** What are the complications of this condition?

**Q4** Would you expect the serum amylase to be elevated here?

**Q5** What is steatorrhoea? How do you confirm the diagnosis? How do you treat this?

**Q6** This patient tells her doctor that she had an episode of haematemesis 3 weeks ago. What is a possible cause in view of her diagnosis?

**Q7** What are the indications for surgery?

## Answers

(A1)
- Calcification likely within the pancreas.
- Changes consistent with chronic pancreatitis.

(A2) Alcohol abuse accounts for 75% of cases.

(A3)
- Abscess.
- Pancreatic pseudocyst: a pseudocyst results from leakage of enzyme-rich pancreatic fluid from a severely inflamed pancreas.
- Fistula.
- Diabetes (type I).
- Biliary tree obstruction with resultant jaundice may be caused by areas of fibrosis.
- Malnutrition and narcotic addiction are more likely to co-exist than actual complications.

(A4) No. Serum amylase is usually normal.

(A5)
- Steatorrhoea is soft, greasy foul-smelling stools.
- Confirmed by 72-hour faecal fat analysis.
- Usually treated with a variable combination of low-fat diets, pancreatic enzymes, antacids and cimetidine.

(A6) Although gastritis and peptic ulcer disease are perhaps more commonly associated with a haematemesis, splenic vein thrombosis with associated varices and hypersplenism should be considered.

(A7) There are no absolute indications, but relative indications include:
- unabating abdominal pain refractory to medical treatment
- biliary obstruction
- suspicion of malignancy.

## Acute pancreatitis

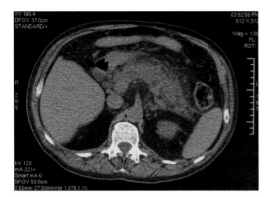

**Figure 2.15**

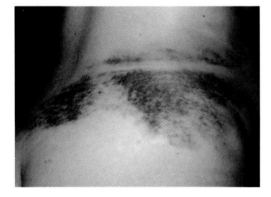

**Figure 2.16**

Figure 2.15 is a CT scan taken from a patient admitted with epigastric pain radiating into his back.

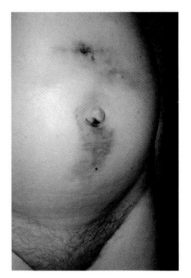

**Figure 2.17**

### Questions

**Q1** What is the diagnosis?

**Q2** What are the causes of this condition?

**Q3** What are the names of the signs being demonstrated in Figures 2.16 and 2.17?

**Q4** What are these two signs associated with and what else may cause flank discoloration?

**Q5** What are Ranson's criteria and how do the indices relate to mortality?

**Q6** What are the principles of treatment?

**Q7** What are the common complications?

**Q8** What is the value of giving a contrast agent during CT scanning?

## Answers

 Acute pancreatitis.

 **Common causes**
Gallstones (45%) and excess alcohol (35%).

**Uncommon causes**
- Idiopathic (10%).
- Ampullary obstruction – pancreatic Ca.
- Hyperlipidaemia.
- Hypercalcaemia.
- Iatrogenic, e.g. ERCP.
- Trauma.
- Congenital: CF, pancreas divisum, cystic disease, haemochromatosis.
- Drugs (thiazide diuretics, histamine, $H_2$ blockers, azathioprine, tetracycline).
- Infections: mumps, coxsackievirus.
- Scorpion bites.

- Grey Turner's sign.
- Cullen's sign: discoloration around umbilicus.

- Severe haemorrhagic pancreatitis.
- Any cause of retroperitoneal bleeding, e.g. AAA rupture.

 These are criteria used to identify high-risk patients with this condition. The factors used are:
- *on presentation*:
  - age >55 years
  - white cell count >16 000 × $10^9$/l
  - rise in blood sugar >11.2 mmol/l
  - LDH >350 mmol/l
  - AST >250mmol/l
- *within 48 hours*:
  - blood urea >1.8 mmol/l rise
  - base deficit >4 mmol/l
  - fall in serum calcium <2.0 mmol/l
  - haematocrit >10% rise
  - $Po_2$ <7.95 kPa
  - third space fluid collection: estimated at >6 l.

Mortality rates associated with numbers of criteria fulfilled are shown in Table 2.1.

**Table 2.1** Mortality rates according to Ranson's criteria

| Number of criteria | Mortality rate (%) |
| --- | --- |
| 0–2 | < 5 |
| 3–4 | 15 |
| 5–6 | 50 |
| 7–8 | 90–100 |

- Hospital admission into surgical ward (mild cases), HDU (moderate severity) or ITU (severe cases).
- iv Fluid resuscitation. Avoid oral fluids. In severe pancreatitis, dehydration leads to reduced splanchnic circulation and pancreatic ischaemia with subsequent necrosis.
- Careful monitoring: urinary catheterisation, pulse oximetry, and central venous pressure monitoring if pancreatitis is severe in an ITU setting. An NG tube should be passed to decompress the stomach and reduce local complications.
- Good analgesia: usually requires morphine although paradoxically this can cause spasm of the sphincter of Oddi.
- Oxygen therapy: to correct hypoxaemia.
- Serial re-assessment. If there is deterioration then CT should be performed to look for necrosis abscess.
- If there is a history of gallstones and USS shows evidence of biliary obstruction, emergency ERCP and sphincterotomy should be performed.
- Deterioration in respiratory function: ITU/HDU setting should be entertained.
- TPN should be considered in severe pancreatitis.
- Patients with severe pancreatitis should be started on broad-spectrum iv antibiotics. In cases of necrotising pancreatitis RCTs have shown a reduction in incidence of sepsis in patients treated with imipenem.

- Shock, pulmonary insufficiency, infection, hypocalcaemia, colonic strictures and pseudocyst formation; 2–10% of patients develop pancreatic pseudocysts. Such patients present with persistent abdominal pain, nausea and vomiting and an abdominal mass. One should wait 6–12 weeks for the pseudocyst to mature before undertaking operative or endoscopic drainage.
- Systemic inflammatory response syndrome (SIRS).
- Multiple organ dysfunction syndrome (MODS).

Computed tomography with contrast allows visualisation and differentiation of healthy perfused parenchyma from patchy poorly perfused necrotic tissue. It is important to differentiate acute pancreatitis from necrotising pancreatitis because the presence and extent of necrosis are key determinants of the clinical course. Seventy per cent of patients with pancreatic necrosis develop infected necrosis. This accounts for 80% of all deaths from pancreatitis and is an indication for surgery.

**Your revision notes:**

# Gastric carcinoma causing gastric outlet obstruction

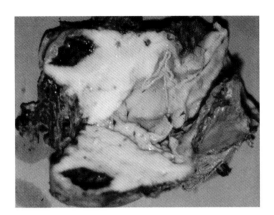

**Figure 2.18**

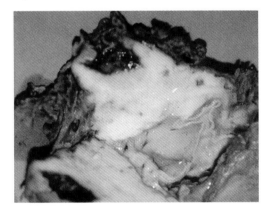

**Figure 2.19**

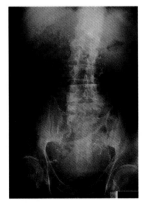

**Figure 2.20**

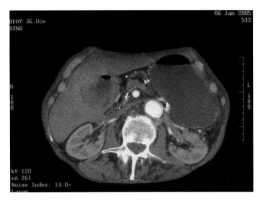

**Figure 2.21**

## Questions

**Q1** Describe what you see in this macroscopic specimen (Figures 2.18 and 2.19). What is the most likely diagnosis when you consider the findings on the plain abdominal film (Figure 2.20) and CT scan (Figure 2.21)?

**Q2** What factors increase the risk of developing this condition?

**Q3** Where in this organ does this disease commonly occur and what is the underlying pathology?

**Q4** How does this disease spread?

**Q5** What is the treatment of this condition?

**Q6** What is the prognosis of this condition?

## Answers

 Stomach.
- This is a macroscopic or gross description of two photos of the same specimen. Gross examination of the distal stomach shows gross thickening consisting of a firm white tumour, with ulceration and obstruction of the pylorus. The tumour is extremely fleshy and firm and has a slight glistening appearance, with a small amount of mucin on the surface. This would be in keeping with an adenocarcinoma, which has caused gastric outlet obstruction.
- AXR + CT show grossly dilated stomach: findings consistent with a gastric outlet obstruction.

- Geographical distribution: high prevalence in the Japanese. Is this diet related? Nitrosamines are thought to be important.
- Genetic factors:
  - family history
  - 4× more common in relatives of patients suffering from the disease than in non-cancer patients. More common in blood group A
  - a small group of patients have a defect of the E-cadherin gene which predisposes them to gastric carcinoma at a young age.
- Pernicious anaemia.
- Chronic atrophic gastritis.
- Gastric polyps.
- Cigarette smoking.
- Gastric ulceration.
- Intestinal metaplasia.
- Post-gastrectomy of the stomach: risk of developing gastric cancer in the remaining part of the stomach is six times that of persons with an intact stomach at 25 years after surgery.
- ? *H. pylori.*

 66% pyloric region; 25% body; 6% cardia; 3% diffuse infiltrating known as linitis plastica. However, these figures are changing. Distribution over the last 10 years is such that there is a gradual decrease in distal cancers and an increase in proximal cancers.

**Pathology**
- *Macroscopically*:
  - polypoid
  - nodular; ulcerating (75%)
  - diffuse infiltrating: causing linitis plastica
  - superficial tumours.
- *Microscopically*:
  - adenocarcinoma
  - well differentiated to anaplastic: typically signet-ring.

 Spread determines ultimate outcome:
- *local*: causing gastric outlet obstruction leading to malnutrition and cachexia
- *lymphatic*: to regional lymph nodes – porta hepatis/coeliac axis
- *transcoelomic*: Kruckenburg tumours in ovary
- *haematogenous*: liver, brain, lung.

Treatment depends on the disease stage:
- palliation is appropriate for patients with distant metastases or unfit for surgical resection
- palliative options include: no surgery, a palliative resection or bypass procedure, a gastrojejunostomy
- curative surgery consists of gastrectomy. The extent of resection is still a matter of debate but a D2 radical gastrectomy seems to offer a survival advantage
- adjuvant chemotherapy.

 Dismal. Once involvement of the regional lymph nodes has occurred 5-year survival falls below 20%.

**Your revision notes:**

# Gallstones

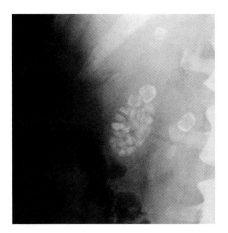

**Figure 2.22**

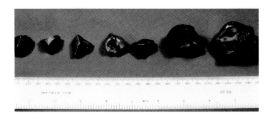

**Figure 2.23**

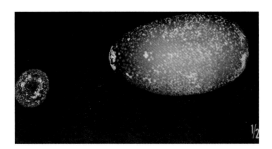

**Figure 2.24**

A 45-year-old obese woman presented to A&E with epigastric pain and vomiting. A plain abdominal radiograph was performed (Figure 2.22).

## Questions

**Q1** What does this radiograph show? What is the likely diagnosis? Is it common to pick this up on a plain abdominal film?

**Q2** What is the prevalence of this condition?

**Q3** What do the photographs in Figures 2.23 and 2.24 depict? What are their chemical compositions?

**Q4** What are the recognised predisposing factors?

**Q5** What is Charcot's triad and of what is it diagnostic?

**Q6** What is Courvoisier's law and what are the exceptions?

**Q7** What are the anatomical boundaries of Calot's triangle? What is its clinical relevance?

## Answers

(A1) • There is a cluster of stones which, in appearance, is consistent with a gallbladder packed with gallstones.
- Three other stones are noted, which are not in close proximity to the former. One is situated fairly superior and may represent a stone lodged in the gallbladder neck.
- Two others appear to be situated more medially and may be impacted in the common bile duct.
- The most likely diagnosis is biliary colic.
- It is not common to see this on a plain film: 10% of cases are evident.

(A2) 10% will have gallstones; only 20% will be symptomatic.

(A3) Gallstones.
- Majority (80%) mixture of cholesterol, bilirubin and calcium (smooth or faceted, light brown and laminated).
- Cholesterol stones (large, pale).
- Pigmented stones (small, black).
- Pathogenesis: related to abnormalities in the relative concentrations of cholesterol, lecithin and bile salts.

(A4) Salmonella typhi, foreign bodies, lipid abnormalities, Crohn's disease, ileal resection, OCP and liver disease. Pigmented stones are associated with haemolytic anaemia, cirrhosis, *E. coli* and *Ascaris lumbricoides*.

(A5) Charcot's triad consists of right upper quadrant pain, jaundice and fever. This is diagnostic of ascending cholangitis.

(A6) In a patient who is jaundiced and has a palpable gallbladder, the obstruction of the common bile duct causing the jaundice is unlikely to be a gallstone. Exceptions to this include a stone occluding the cystic duct and a synchronous obstruction of the distal CBD.

(A7) The liver, common hepatic duct and the cystic duct. During cholecystectomy, the cystic artery and its branches are found running through Calot's triangle.

# Common bile duct stones

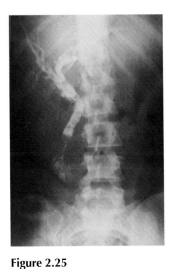

**Figure 2.25**

A 50-year-old woman presented with jaundice following a laparoscopic cholecystectomy.

## Questions

**Q1** What is the diagnosis?

**Q2** What does this radiograph show? What is the diagnosis?

**Q3** What procedure has this patient undergone and what main complications would she have been told about beforehand?

**Q4** What are the other treatment options?

## Answers

(A1) • Retained CBD stone (15% of those with gallstones).

(A2) • A stent is noted in the common bile duct.
• Several filling defects are detected, consistent with common bile duct stones.

(A3) ERCP + sphincterotomy + stenting.
• Morbidity of ERCP is <10%, mortality 1%.
• Main complications are: cholangitis, haemorrhage, pancreatitis and perforation.

(A4) • Open exploration of the CBD.
• Open or laparoscopic choledochoscopy and stone extraction.
• Dissolution therapy.
• Lithotripsy.

## Small bowel obstruction

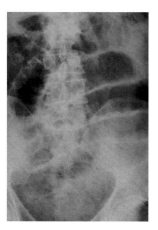

**Figure 2.26**

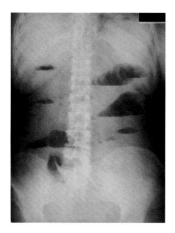

**Figure 2.27**

## Questions

**Q1** What does this abdominal X-ray show (Figure 2.26)? What are the distinguishing features? If you could persuade a reluctant radiographer to do an erect AXR (Figure 2.27), what would that film show?

**Q2** How would a patient with this problem present?

**Q3** What are the common causes?

**Q4** How would you manage a patient with this condition if he presented to A&E?

**Q5** Are there any clinical features that you would consider suggest actual or impending intestinal ischaemia?

## Answers

- This is a supine AXR, which shows dilated small bowel loops.
- Small bowel is recognised by its central position and valvulae conniventes in the proximal small bowel. These are not present in the terminal ileum.
- An erect AXR would show the distended loops stacked in a ladder pattern but would also readily demonstrate air/fluid levels in the distended gut (Figure 2.27).

- Central colicky abdominal pain.
- Vomiting.
- Constipation (usually a late sign).
- Abdominal distension.

- Intra-abdominal adhesions from previous operations (70%).
- Herniae.
- Abdominal malignancy.
- *Causes*: divide into luminal, gut wall, extrinsic.

**Luminal**
- Foreign bodies.
- Bezoars.
- Worm infection.
- Gallstone.
- Meconium in the neonate.

**Gut wall**
- Atresia.
- Strictures from Crohn's disease or TB.
- Tumours, which are often lymphomas or GIST.

**Extrinsic**
- Adhesions.
- Herniae.
- Volvulus.
- Intussusception.
- Congenital bands.
- Neoplasms.

Usual history and examination are needed to find underlying cause.

**Treatment**
Initially conservative expecting relief of symptoms by:
- NG tube with regular aspiration
- catheterisation: to closely monitor input and urine output. These patients are often dehydrated on admission
- nil by mouth regime
- anti-emetics
- analgesia
- iv fluids.

Treat underlying cause:
- most SBO due to adhesions will settle with conservative measures
- if there is an obvious hernia, operate and repair
- if this is a virgin abdomen lower the threshold to operate
- need to consider the possibility of underlying ischaemic bowel (blood gases), then, if suspected, surgical intervention is required
- if conservative measures fail (trial usually 48 hours) then need to consider an operation. Trial of 5 days with drip and suck from the multicentric studies does not seem to increase complications in those who eventually progress to surgery
- serial examination of the patient is important to look for deterioration.

- Features of strangulation are continuous unremitting pain and severe pain only partially relieved or unrelieved by opiate analgesics. On examination, the degree of tachycardia, tenderness, localised tenderness and peritonism are the most important signs to look for.
- Determine whether the loops of small bowel on X-ray correspond to the area of maximal tenderness.
- There is usually a combination of features rather than a single finding that suggests ischaemia.
- If small bowel is grossly dilated the risks of perforation and ischaemia are high.
- If there is evidence of a closed loop obstruction the patient requires an urgent laparotomy, as the risk of strangulation and perforation is greater.
- Look at WCC: greater than $20 \times 10^9/l$ indicates that ischaemia is more likely.

**Your revision notes:**

## Meckel's diverticulum

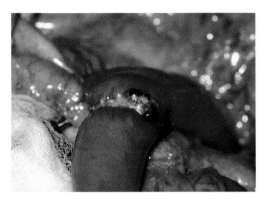

**Figure 2.28**

This lesion was found in the distal ileum at laparotomy for small bowel obstruction.

## Questions

(Q1) What is it?

(Q2) How else may it present?

(Q3) If this lesion was found to be inflamed during appendicectomy, how should it be dealt with?

(Q4) If the lesion were not inflamed would your management be any different?

(Q5) Describe its embryological origin.

## Answers

(A1) A Meckel's diverticulum.

(A2)
- Haemorrhage: one-sixth of Meckel's contain ectopic gastric mucosa capable of acid secretion, which can cause peptic ulceration leading to bleeding. This is the most common cause of lower gastrointestinal bleeding in the paediatric population.
- Obstruction: a remnant band joining the tip of the diverticulum to the umbilicus may be the focus around which the small bowel twists and obstructs.
- Perforation: ectopic gastric acid secretion can lead to ulceration and perforation downstream of the Meckel's.
- Diverticulitis: obstruction of a narrow neck may result in an acute inflammation which may be clinically indistinguishable from acute appendicitis.
- Intussusception: the diverticulum may invert and become the focal point of an intussusception – presents as intestinal obstruction.
- Littre's hernia (rare): Meckel's diverticulum is present in an inguinal or femoral hernia.

(A3) Resected with a short segment of adjacent normal bowel and a primary anastomosis is performed.

(A4) If it was non-inflamed it should be left alone. However some surgeons may elect to resect a normal-looking Meckel's diverticulum if it had a particularly narrow neck that may later obstruct.

(A5) This is a true diverticulum that is an embryological remnant of the vitellointestinal duct. It is said to be present in 2% of the population, 2 inches long and sited 2 feet from the ileocaecal valve on the antimesenteric border of the ileum. It becomes inflamed in 2% of the population.

## Gastrointestinal stromal tumours (GIST)

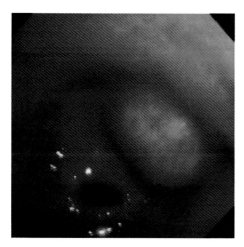

**Figure 2.29**

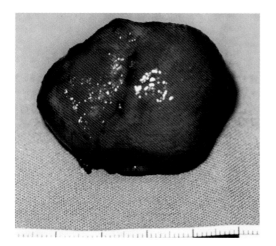

**Figure 2.30**

A 60-year-old lady presented with vague upper abdominal pain. Figure 2.29 shows the finding from an upper GI endoscopy; Figure 2.30 shows the specimen removed at the time of surgery.

### Questions

**Q1** What is the most likely diagnosis?

**Q2** What is the epidemiology of this condition?

**Q3** How does this condition present?

**Q4** What is the treatment of this condition?

**Q5** What is Carney's triad?

**Q6** Give two prognostic features of the disease that predict clinical behaviour.

## Answers

(A1) Gastrointestinal stromal tumour (GIST).

(A2) • Peak incidence 50–70 years.
• Males and females equally affected.
• Most common site is the stomach.

(A3) • Gastric stromal tumours are a common incidental finding at autopsy but only a small proportion are symptomatic. Most common presenting features are those of upper gastrointestinal haemorrhage (up to 90%) with haematemesis, malaena and anaemia.
• Other symptoms include epigastric pain, weight loss and presence of a palpable mass.
• Incidental finding at time of laparotomy or gastroscopy.

(A4) Surgical excision with a 2 cm margin of surrounding tissue. Biological behaviour is difficult to predict but in general the larger the tumour the greater the number of mitoses and degree of cellular atypia, and therefore the more malignant.

(A5) • It is important to recognise that these tumours may be part of clinical syndromes.
• Carney's triad = extra-adrenal paraganglioma, pulmonary chondroma, gastric stromal tumours. Affects young women. Can be diagnosed if two out of three features present.

(A6) Size of the tumour, mitotic index and whether C-kit protein positive. Also whether completely resected at operation.

## Porcelain gallbladder

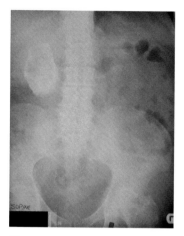

**Figure 2.31**

### Questions

**Q1** What does this AXR demonstrate? What is its significance?

**Q2** What are the aetiology and pathology of this condition?

**Q3** How do these patients normally present?

**Q4** How would you investigate this patient?

**Q5** How would you manage a patient with this disease?

## Answers

 A calcified or 'porcelain' gallbladder. This is a pre-malignant condition for developing carcinoma of the gallbladder (GB).

- 90% of patients with GB cancer have gallstones.
- GB cancer increased by 15-fold 20 years after surgery for gastric ulcer.
- Chronic inflammation due to typhoid appears to carry an increased risk.
- There are high-risk ethnic groups: South West American Indians. High incidence of the anomalous common bile duct and pancreatic duct junction noted.
- Mostly mucus-secreting adenocarcinomas (90%); 10% squamous in nature.
- Rare. F:M = 4:1.
- Spread to liver, either directly or via the portal vein.
- Staging and grading are based on Nevin:
  - *grade I–III*: well, moderately or poorly differentiated
  - *stage I*: confined to the mucosa and via lymphatics to the porta hepatis
  - *stage II*: breaches the muscularis mucosae
  - *stage III*: extends through the muscularis propria
  - *stage IV*: additionally involves the cystic node
  - *stage V*: involvement of the liver or other organs – usually segment IV or V in the gallbladder bed.
- Nevin's score = grade + stage: directly affects survival. No patient in his series with a score of >6 survived one year.
- Generally 5-year survival is less than 5%.

- Peak age of incidence is 70–75 years. May be silent for a long time and the commonest diagnosis is made post-operatively in GBs removed for stone disease. Can be a problem in this day of laparoscopic cholecystectomy because of the risk of tumour implantation at the extraction port.
- Symptomatic cancers may present with biliary obstruction – jaundice, acute cholecystitis or empyema of the gallbladder.

- Laboratory tests: non-specific.
- USS: may suggest a mass.
- Confirm with CT.
- ERCP/PTC: involvement of the duct of segment V by a GB mass is highly suggestive of cancer.
- Endoscopic USS.

- Prophylactic cholecystectomy for asymptomatic stones except in the case of a porcelain GB is not indicated as the risks outweigh the benefits.
- Treatment depends on staging and mode of presentation and fitness of patient.
- Once carcinoma of the GB has invaded the hilar ducts and caused obstructive jaundice it is rarely resectable.
- If well-localised: wedge resection of the GB bed or formal excision of segments IV and V should be considered.
- Generally results are poor. Patients should be palliated and treated by stenting if jaundiced.
- Adjuvant therapy: external beam radiotherapy has been reported by some to be of benefit. GB cancer is regarded as chemo-resistant.

# Small bowel diverticulosis

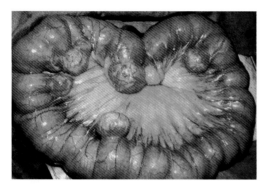

**Figure 2.32**

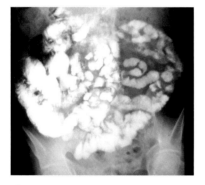

**Figure 2.33**

## Questions

**Q1** What is the diagnosis?

**Q2** What are the common sites of occurrence?

**Q3** What is the aetiology?

**Q4** What are the usual associated symptoms?

**Q5** How do you treat them?

## Answers

(A1) Small bowel diverticulosis.

(A2) Almost half of the diverticulae occur in the duodenum; 25% are Meckel's diverticulum. Jejuno-ileal diverticulae are less common and the majority (80%) occur in the jejunum.

(A3) They can be congenital or acquired. The acquired ones result from intestinal dyskinesis and occur as herniations along the sites of entry of blood vessels.

(A4) They are usually asymptomatic. They may sometimes present with symptoms of malabsorption, bleeding, diverticulitis, perforation and obstruction. An enterolith may rarely form in the diverticulum, which can then obstruct the lumen.

(A5) Asymptomatic incidental diverticulae do not require any treatment. Symptomatic jejuno-ileal diverticulae require limited resection and anastomosis. Symptomatic duodenal diverticulae require diverticulectomy.

# Pancreatic pseudocyst

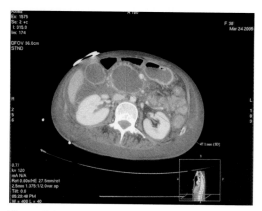

**Figure 2.34**

Figures 2.34 and 2.35 show an abdominal CT scan of a 65-year-old male 5 weeks after an attack of acute pancreatitis.

## Questions

**Q1**  What do the CT scans show? Why is it so called?

**Q2**  What are the clinical symptoms associated with this? How do you investigate this?

**Q3**  What possible complications can this lead to?

**Q4**  How is it treated?

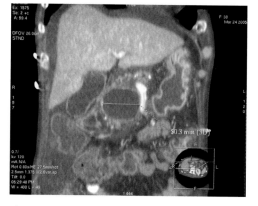

**Figure 2.35**

## Answers

**(A1)** The CT scans demonstrate a large pseudocyst in the body of the pancreas. It is of homogeneous density with a well-defined wall. It is compressing the stomach anteriorly. It is termed a pseudocyst as the wall lacks an epithelial lining and is enclosed by fibrous or granulation tissue. Therefore it is not a true cyst.

**(A2)** Abdominal pain, vomiting, jaundice, fever. The signs include a palpable epigastric mass which may be tender. Pyrexia, jaundice and anaemia may be present. Investigations include blood tests, which may reveal raised white cells, low Hb, abnormal LFTs, and elevated serum amylase (in 50% of patients). Abdominal ultrasound and CT scan are very helpful in diagnosis and follow-up. An ERCP is helpful in chronic pseudocysts with associated bile duct or pancreatic duct abnormalities.

**(A3)** Infection, rupture, bleeding, obstruction of bile duct, stomach or duodenum.

**(A4)** 
- Treatment is recommended for cysts persisting for more than six weeks or larger than 6 cm in size.
- The procedure of choice is internal drainage into the stomach (cystogastrostomy) or into a roux-en-Y loop of jejunum (cystojejunostomy) and rarely into the duodenum (cystoduodenostomy). This can be achieved by an open operation, laparoscopic operation or by endoscopy. Percutaneous drainage is indicated for infected and extra-anatomical pseudocysts.

# Splenomegaly

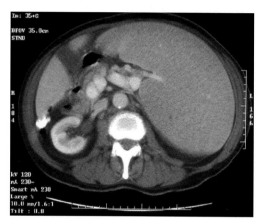

**Figure 2.36**

## Questions

**Q1** Identify the organ enlarged on this CT scan. What are its functions?

**Q2** Name five causes for its enlargement.

**Q3** What are the indications for removal of this organ?

**Q4** What investigations are carried out to evaluate injury to this?

**Q5** What are the different methods of management of injury to this?

**Q6** What are the post-operative complication after this?

**Q7** What are the long-term precautions to be taken?

## Answers

**A1** Spleen. The functions of the spleen can be listed as:
- *immune functions*: major site of IgM production. It is also involved in processing of foreign antigen and synthesis of opsonins, tuftsins and properdin
- *filter functions*: removal of effete RBCs and platelets. Removal of iron from the ingested degraded haemoglobin by culling and returning to plasma. It also removes non-cellular material like bacteria, especially pneumococci
- *pitting functions*: particulate inclusions are removed from the RBCs and the repaired cells are returned back into the circulation. The inclusions removed include Howell–Jolly bodies and Heinz bodies
- *reservoir functions*: the spleen contains roughly 8% of the red cell mass. An enlarged spleen may contain an even larger proportion
- *cytopoiesis*: haemopoiesis during intra-uterine life. Proliferation of T and B cells and macrophages following antigenic challenge. This proliferation is also seen in myeloproliferative disorders, thalassaemias and chronic haemolytic anaemias.

**A2** There are numerous causes of splenic enlargement:
- *infective*: bacterial (typhoid, paratyphoid, typhus, splenic abscess), spirochaetal (Weil's disease, syphilis), viral (infectious mononucleosis, HIV), protozoal/parasitic (malaria, kala-azar, hydatid cyst, schistosomiasis)
- *blood diseases*: acute leukaemia, chronic leukaemia, ITP, hereditary spherocytosis, auto-immune haemolytic anaemia, sickle cell disease
- *metabolic*: rickets, amyloid, porphyria, Gaucher's disease
- *circulatory*: infarct, portal hypertension
- *collagen disease*: Still's disease, Felty syndrome
- *neoplastic*: angioma, Hodgkin's lymphoma, myelofibrosis.

**A3** The indications for splenectomy include:
- *trauma*: accidental, operative
- *blood disorders*: hereditary spherocytosis, ITP, hypersplenism
- *oncological*: part of en-bloc resection, diagnostic, therapeutic
- portal hypertension
- hydatid cyst
- splenic abscess
- splenic artery aneurysm.

**A4** Abdominal ultrasound, CT scan, diagnostic peritoneal lavage.

**A5** Conservative management, splenectomy with or without auto-transplantation, partial splenectomy, splenorrhaphy.

**A6** Bleeding, gastric injuries, sub-phrenic collection, prolonged gastric atony, chest infection, acute gastric dilatation, pancreatic injuries/fistula, infections.

**A7**
- Precautions against opportunist post-splenectomy infection (OPSI).
- Prophylactic antibiotics (penicillin) and vaccination (*pneumococcus, H. influezae* and *meningococcus*).

## Subphrenic abscess

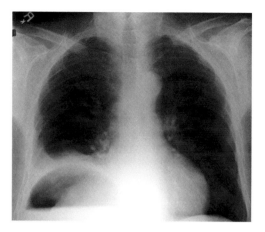

**Figure 2.37**

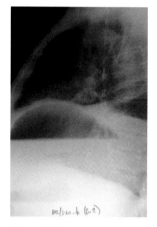

**Figure 2.38**

A 78-year-old gentleman was admitted with rigors and sweats two weeks following a Hartmann's procedure for perforated diverticular disease. He had also noticed that he had been experiencing persistent hiccups. These X-rays were taken on admission.

## Questions

**Q1** What does the CXR show and in view of his history what is the most likely diagnosis?

**Q2** What other causes can you think of that may also cause this problem?

**Q3** What other symptoms or signs may this patient demonstrate? What other features may the CXR show in this condition?

**Q4** What is the microbiology of this condition?

**Q5** Name two other imaging modalities that may help confirm the diagnosis.

**Q6** What is the treatment of choice for this problem?

## Answers

**(A1)**
- CXR shows an air–fluid level below the right hemidiaphragm.
- Subphrenic abscess: the subphrenic spaces are the most common sites for the development of intra-abdominal abscesses. In septic post-operative surgical patients it is very important to consider subphrenic abscess as a possibility after pulmonary, urinary and pelvic sepsis have been excluded.
- Remember 'pus somewhere, pus nowhere, pus under the diaphragm'.

**(A2)** Spontaneous abdominal organ perforation, peptic ulcer disease, appendicitis, diverticular disease, Crohn's disease, cholecystitis, intestinal infarction and penetrating abdominal injuries.

**(A3)**
- Patient usually looks unwell with anorexia, nausea, upper abdominal pain/back pain radiating to shoulder tip. Hiccups – due to diaphragmatic irritation. Swinging pyrexia and tachycardia.
- CXR may show elevation of the hemidiaphragm, pleural effusion.

**(A4)** Usually polymicrobial: Gram-negative and anaerobes.

**(A5)**
- USS and/or CT.
- USS more commonly employed: no ionising radiation, portable and can easily be performed in the ITU setting on a ventilated patient if necessary.

**(A6)** Treatment of choice is percutaneous drainage ideally under imaging guidance (USS/CT) with appropriate intravenous antibiotic therapy. Surgical drainage is performed only if patients have failed to respond to percutaneous drainage or in those abscesses not amenable to percutaneous drainage.

## Pseudomyxoma peritonei

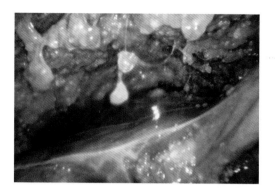

**Figure 2.39**

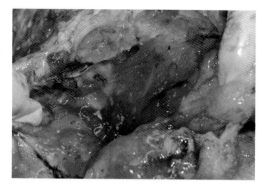

**Figure 2.42**

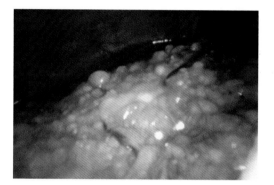

**Figure 2.40**

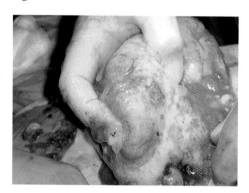

**Figure 2.43**

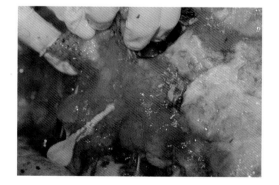

**Figure 2.41**

A 54-year-old female presented with gradually increasing abdominal size for the past six months associated with vague abdominal discomfort. Laparotomy revealed a jelly-like substance widely disseminated in the abdomen.

### Questions

**Q1** What is the diagnosis?

**Q2** What are the usual aetiological factors?

**Q3** What are the different clinical presentations?

**Q4** How do you manage this condition?

**Q5** Is this malignant? What is the prognosis?

## Answers

 Pseudomyxoma peritonei. This is a rare condition characterised by copious production of mucinous ascites that eventually fills up the peritoneal cavity ('jelly belly').

 The most common structure of origin is the appendix. It may also originate in the ovary in many females. The other organs of origin are colon, rectum, stomach, gallbladder, bile ducts, small intestine and lungs.

- Increasing abdominal size.
- Features associated with raised intra-abdominal pressure: bloating.
- Reflux, new onset hernia and utero-vaginal prolapse.
- Symptoms mimicking acute appendicitis.
- Palpable abdominal lump.
- Vague abdominal pain.
- Systemic symptoms: anorexia, weight loss.

- Contrast-enhanced CT scan and MRI are helpful and show small bowel central compartmentalisation with omental caking. Tumour markers CA 19.9 and CA 125 are frequently elevated. Anaemia is not uncommon.
- Debulking procedures: removal of as much of the mucinous tumour as possible with some limited resectional procedures such as right hemicolectomy, omentectomy, hysterectomy and bilateral oophorectomy.
- Complete cyto reduction: requires proper patient selection and involves six peritonectomy procedures (Sugarbaker) with no tumour deposit more than 2.5 mm left behind. Extensive operation associated with significant morbidity and 3–5% mortality.
- Non-surgical methods: possible beneficial role for Cox 2 inhibitors.
- Intra-peritoneal chemotherapy: can penetrate nodules up to 2–3 mm in size. Usual agents are mitomycin C and 5-fluoro-uracil. Heated intra-operative intra-peritoneal chemotherapy (the Coliseum technique) has been tried.

 This is best considered as a borderline malignancy. This consists of a spectrum of pathological entities ranging from benign to invasive malignancy. It is divided into three broad groups: disseminated, peritoneal adenomucinosis, peritoneal mucinous carcinomatosis and an intermediate hybrid group. Maximal surgical cytoreduction and adjuvant chemotherapy can achieve 5-year survival rates of 86%. The average 5-year survival is about 50%.

# Free gas under the diaphragm/pneumoperitoneum

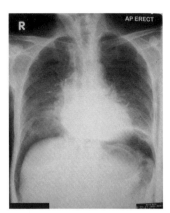

**Figure 2.44**

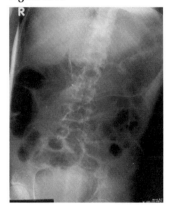

**Figure 2.45**

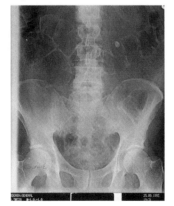

**Figure 2.46**

These radiographs (Figures 2.44–2.46) were taken of a 34-year-old gentleman with a 24-hour history of sudden-onset worsening generalised abdominal pain.

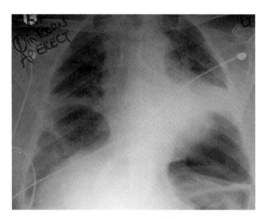

**Figure 2.47**

## Questions

**Q1** What do Figures 2.44–2.46 show?

**Q2** What is the most likely diagnosis?

**Q3** Are the findings shown on these radiographs invariably present in this surgical emergency?

**Q4** What are the typical presenting features of this condition? What do you understand by the term right paracolic gutter phenomenon?

**Q5** How would you manage this patient?

**Q6** What are the other potential complications of this disease?

**Q7** Who are affected by this condition and what are the predisposing factors?

**Q8** How much free air needs to be present to be detected on CXR?

**Q9** Look at Figure 2.47. This subsequent CXR was taken the same day on a 60-year-old gentleman for investigation of acute abdominal pain. Is there free gas present here too?

**Q10** What other conditions may mimic the appearance of a pneumoperitoneum?

## Answers

**A1**
- Free air under both diaphragms (Figure 2.44).
- Visible falciform ligament (Figure 2.45).
- Riggler's sign: the bowel wall can be seen due to free intraperitoneal air (Figures 2.45 and 2.46).

**A2** In a gentleman of this age and with this story, the most likely diagnosis is a perforated peptic ulcer, probably a duodenal ulcer.

**A3** No. Free air under the diaphragm is only present in about 70% of cases of perforated peptic ulcer disease. The other findings are less commonly present.

**A4** Typically perforated duodenal ulcers produce acute-onset epigastric pain followed by more generalised abdominal pain. Sometimes right iliac fossa occurs due to duodenal gastric contents accumulating at this site under gravity. This can sometimes be confused with acute appendicitis. This tracking of leaking fluids leading to symptoms at a different area is called right paracolic gutter phenomenon. The patient may also complain of right shoulder tip pain due to referred pain from diaphragmatic irritation. Nausea is common but vomiting is uncommon. Examination reveals a distended and 'boardlike' abdomen due to involuntary contraction of the rectus abdominis. There is a paucity/absence of bowel sounds. Systemic signs include pyrexia, tachycardia, tachypnoea and a dry tongue.

**A5** Surgery in most cases.

**Surgery**
Most surgeons would advocate laparotomy and oversewing of the ulcer with placement of an omental patch over the site of the ulcer. Some would combine this with a definitive procedure such as truncal vagotomy or highly selective vagotomy. More radical surgery may be indicated in large perforations not amenable to primary closure.

**Conservative**
If patient is a high-risk candidate for surgery and clinically has no or minimal peritoneal signs consider conservative treatment. This is with strict NBM with iv fluids and iv antibiotics and passage of an NG tube and urine catheter for strict input/output. Opiate analgesia is given. The patient needs to be serially examined and closely monitored. If there is any sign of clinical deterioration surgery is indicated.

**A6** Obstruction, fistulation and haemorrhage.

**A7** DU – young males below 50 years, smokers, alcohol, use of steroids, NSAIDs.

**A8** 1 ml.

**A9** No. This is Chilaiditi's syndrome: presence of intestine (colon) between the liver and diaphragm.

**A10** Subphrenic abscess, pulmonary collapse, subdiaphragmatic fat and cysts in pneumatosis intestinalis.

## CLO test

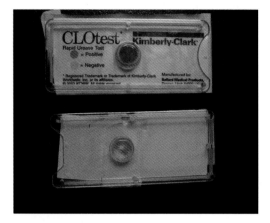

**Figure 2.48**

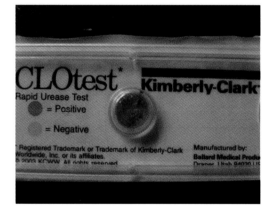

**Figure 2.49**

A 38-year-old female presented with upper abdominal pain and dyspepsia. An OGD was done which revealed antral gastritis. A further test was done on the mucosa and the findings are shown.

### Questions

**Q1** What is the purpose of this test? What is the underlying reaction involved in this test?

**Q2** What are the various methods of detecting this organism?

**Q3** How do you treat this?

**Q4** What is the worrying condition this organism has been linked to?

## Answers

 This is the CLO test to demonstrate the presence of *Helicobacter pylori* in the mucosa of the stomach. The underlying reaction is the ability of the organism to hydrolyse urea with the formation of ammonia, a strong alkali.

 • CLO test: urease kit test on gastric mucosal biopsies.
• Histology: Giemsa stains.
• Culture of *H. pylori*.
• Serological tests.
• Urea breath test.

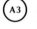 Combined antibiotic treatment regimen usually for two weeks. It commonly includes a proton pump blocker (e.g. omeprezole) and two antibiotics such as metronidazole (or tinidazole) and amoxicillin (or clarythromycin). Eradication rates of around 90% can be achieved.

 *H. pylori* is presently classified as a class 1 carcinogen, because of its association with carcinoma of the stomach.

# Section 3

# Vascular

# Acute ischaemia of the lower limb

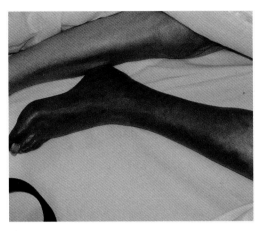

**Figure 3.1**

## Questions

Q1  What is the diagnosis?

Q2  What are the presenting features of this condition?

Q3  What are the causes of this problem?

Q4  What is the treatment of this condition?

Q5  How is thrombus distinguished from embolus in acute ischaemia?

## Answers

 Critical ischaemia of the left leg.

 Learn the six 'P's:
- pain
- pallor
- pulselessness
- paraesthesia
- paralysis
- perishing cold.

- Embolic: most commonly arise from the following sites:
  - heart: left ventricular mural thrombus following acute myocardial infarction and congestive cardiac failure; from the left atrium in atrial fibrillation
  - peripheral blood vessels: aortic or popliteal aneurysm, iliofemoral stenoses.
- Acute thrombosis of an already atherosclerotic segment of artery.

It is often difficult to make the distinction in the lower limb.

 *Medical treatment*; liaise with medical colleagues:
- treat atrial fibrillation, e.g. with digoxin after confirmation with ECG
- treatment of arterial embolism: intravenous analgesia and heparinisation
- emergency angiogram +/– thrombolysis (with streptokinase or tissue plasminogen activator) if there are no facilities to do so
- this should be followed by heparinisation and commencement of warfarin for at least six months
- further cardiac investigations such as echocardiogram.

*Surgical option* would be femoral embolectomy.

The choice between the two therapies depends on the degree of the ischaemia:
- patients who have developed paralysis or paraesthesia of the limb should proceed to embolectomy, as there may be significant delay to reperfusion when the time taken for angiography and thrombolysis is taken into account
- patient should be consented for amputation if the leg becomes unsalvageable.

 Can be complicated especially in lower limb.

Findings suggestive of embolus include no prior history of vascular disease, normal contralateral leg circulation, history of cardiac arrhythmia or recent myocardial infarction. Patients with embolic disease frequently have profound leg ischaemia due to the proximal nature of the occlusion (aortic or femoral bifurcation) and the absence of developed collaterals. Occasionally angiography may be required to distinguish between the two.

## Charcot's foot

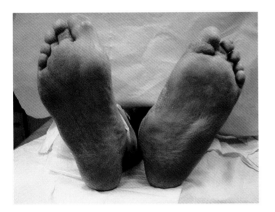

**Figure 3.2**

### Questions

(Q1) What abnormality is shown here in this 48-year-old diabetic patient?

(Q2) What is the underlying pathology?

(Q3) How can the diagnosis be confirmed?

(Q4) How is this condition managed?

(Q5) What other diabetic complications are likely in these patients?

## Answers

(A1) Charcot deformity of the left foot.

(A2) Elevated bone turnover with net bone resorption and destruction, increased vascularity.

(A3) Bone scan plus white cell scan; MRI.

(A4) Immobilisation and pressure relief often with a cast (air cast, total contact cast). Pamidronate infusions may be beneficial, but the evidence for this is controversial.

(A5) Neuropathy, retinopathy, nephropathy.

## Infected femoral pseudoaneurysm

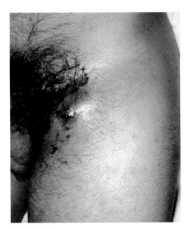

**Figure 3.3**

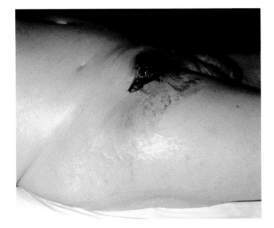

**Figure 3.4**

These two pictures show the groins of two young drug addicts who presented to the A&E department with these painful lesions.

### Questions

Q1 What is your diagnosis?

Q2 What are the likely infecting organisms?

Q3 What would be your initial management?

Q4 What are the principles of operative surgery for this condition?

Q5 What vascular reconstruction is required?

## Answers

(A1) Infected femoral pseudoaneurysm: although it could be a simple abscess it is dangerous to assume this in a drug addict who is using the femoral vessels for injections.

(A2) Classically, arterial infections are associated with *Staphylococcus aureus, Streptococcus viridans,* and *Salmonella.* In this setting however a wide range of Gram-negative organisms could also be involved.

(A3) • Establish ABC, with emphasis on gaining venous access and cross-matching blood to support the circulation in case rupture and bleeding should occur.
• Baseline inflammatory markers, hepatitis B and HIV status.
• Commence high-dose, broad-spectrum systemic antibiotics.
• Confirm diagnosis with ultrasound +/– angiography.
• Prepare for theatre.

(A4) • Gain vascular control.
• Thorough debridement of all necrotic infected tissue, including femoral vessels if necessary.
• Ligation of vessels proximally and distally.

(A5) Vascular reconstruction is required if the limb is threatened by ischaemia after vessel ligation. Prosthetic graft material should be avoided because of the risk of graft infection. Vein from the opposite leg should be used. Frequently, the common femoral artery can be ligated without reconstruction, and the limb will remain viable. The risk of the patient infecting or damaging the graft and re-presenting with bleeding is high in drug abusers.

# Ankle brachial pressure index (ABPI)

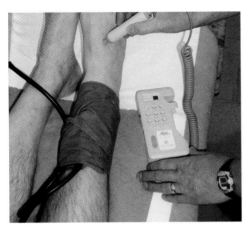

**Figure 3.5**

## Questions

Q1 What investigation is this?

Q2 What is a normal result for this investigation?

Q3 What result would you expect in a patient with critical limb ischaemia?

Q4 When is this investigation unreliable?

Q5 What alternative vascular laboratory investigations can be used instead to measure limb ischaemia?

## Answers

(A1) Ankle systolic pressure measurement/ankle brachial pressure ratio (ABPI).

(A2) ABPI $\geq$ 1.0.

(A3) ABPI < 0.5 or ankle pressure < 50 mmHg.

(A4) In the presence of calcified calf vessels, particularly in diabetic patients.

(A5) Toe pressure measurements, pole test Doppler, transcutaneous oximetry.

# Ischaemic finger

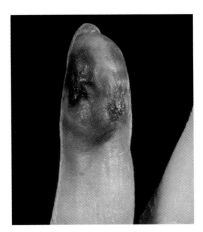

**Figure 3.6**

This 42-year-old woman presented with a two-day history of a painful finger.

## Questions

**Q1** What is the differential diagnosis?

**Q2** What investigations would you perform?

**Q3** What is your initial management?

**Q4** Why does pressure from a cervical rib cause this condition?

**Q5** What complication can occur after surgery to relieve this compression?

## Answers

 • Embolism.
• Digital artery thrombosis.
• Vasculitis.

 • Vasculitic/thrombophilic/hyperviscosity blood tests.
• ECG: evidence of atrial fibrillation?
• CXR plus thoracic inlet views for cervical rib.
• Echocardiogram looking for a source of embolism.
• Duplex/angiography.

 • Analgesia.
• Heparin infusion.

 Chronic subclavian artery stenosis with post-stenotic dilatation and aneurysm formation. Thrombus in the aneurysm embolises to the digits.

 • Brachial plexus injury.
• Phrenic nerve injury.
• Horner's syndrome.
• Pneumothorax.
• Haemothorax.

# Varicose veins with ulcer

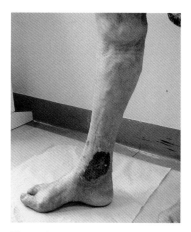

**Figure 3.7**

## Questions

**Q1** What is the likely aetiology of this ulcer?

**Q2** What investigations would you perform?

**Q3** How would you get this ulcer to heal?

**Q4** What are the success rates of bandaging?

**Q5** Name five other causes of leg ulceration.

## Answers

 Venous ulcer, typical site and appearance, associated varicose veins.

- ABPI.
- Venous duplex scan.

 If ABPI > 0.8 and deep veins are patent, apply compression bandaging over dressings. Treat any sepsis. Consider superficial venous surgery for:
- non-healing ulcer despite bandaging
- frequent recurrence
- inability to tolerate bandaging
- superficial venous incompetence alone, or segmental deep reflux; not for complete deep reflux and post-thrombotic deep reflux.

 75% healed at 6 months, 25% recurrence rates.

- Arterial (ischaemic) ulcers.
- Vasculitic ulcers (rheumatoid).
- Pyoderma gangrenosum.
- Necrobiosis lipoidica/diabetes.
- Skin malignancy.
- Chronic sepsis.
- Haematological disorders (sickle cell disease).

# Popliteal aneurysm

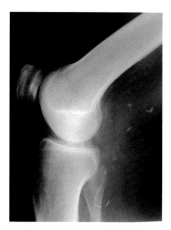

**Figure 3.8**

## Questions

**Q1** What does this plain X-ray film show?

**Q2** Name three ways in which this lesion can present with symptoms.

**Q3** What other investigations would you perform?

**Q4** At what size would you plan to repair this lesion?

**Q5** What are the treatment options?

## Answers

**(A1)** Calcified popliteal artery with aneurysm.

**(A2)**
- Distal embolism.
- Rupture.
- Compression (DVT, knee pain).

**(A3)**
- Angiogram to assess run off, plan for repair of larger aneurysm.
- Abdominal USS to look for AAA (30% incidence).

**(A4)** >2.5 cm or when symptomatic.

**(A5)**
- Ligation and bypass with either vein or prosthetic graft.
- *In situ* repair with inlay graft.
- Endovascular stent graft.

# Superficial femoral artery obstruction

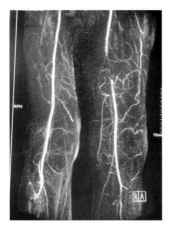

**Figure 3.9**

## Questions

**Q1** What abnormality is shown here?

**Q2** What is the likely aetiology?

**Q3** What are the five main risk factors for this disease?

**Q4** In the presence of limb-threatening ischaemia how would you manage this patient?

**Q5** What are the endovascular success rates for treating such a lesion? What are the surgical success rates?

## Answers

(A1) Occlusion of left SFA in its mid-segment. Approximately 5 cm in length. Also poor run off in calf with disease on both sides.

(A2) Multilevel disease, with collaterals, indicates that this is a chronic atherosclerotic occlusion. Acute thrombo-embolism would not give these appearances.

(A3) 
- Smoking.
- Diabetes.
- Hypertension.
- Hyperlipidaemia.
- Family history.

(A4) 
- Optimise medical condition (diabetes, BP, treat sepsis etc).
- Attempt percutaneous angioplasty either luminal or subintimal.
- No evidence for the benefit of routine stenting in the femoral popliteal segment.
- If PTA fails, work up for a femoro-popliteal bypass graft.

(A5) 
- PTA success for 5 cm SFA occlusion 70% patency 3 years, 50% at 5 years.
- Femoral above-knee (A-K) popliteal vein graft patency 80% 3 years, 70% 5 years.
- Femoral above-knee (A-K) popliteal prosthetic graft patency 70% 3 years, 50% 5 years.

## Diabetic foot

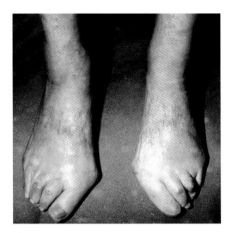

**Figure 3.10**

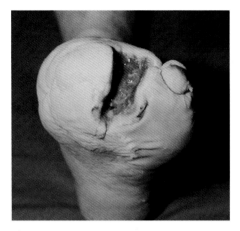

**Figure 3.13**

A 65-year-old male, a known diabetic for 20 years, presented with these evolving foot problems following a trivial injury.

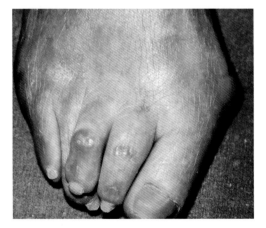

**Figure 3.11**

## Questions

Q1) What is the term given to this problem?

Q2) What are the underlying abnormalities?

Q3) What are the usual triggering factors?

Q4) What are the different clinical symptoms? What is a Charcot's joint?

Q5) How do you manage this?

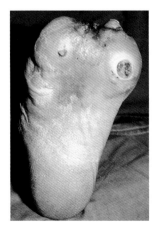

**Figure 3.12**

## Answers

 Diabetic foot.

 This is a risk in all long-standing diabetics and the lifetime risk of foot ulceration in these patients is 15%. Diabetes is still the leading cause of non-traumatic major amputation today. The three underlying factors are:
- neuropathy
- large vessel and small vessel ischaemic disease
- infection.

Neuropathy affects about 20–40% of diabetics within 20 years of diagnosis. This leads to a 'glove and stocking' sensorimotor neuropathy and consequent foot joint deformities.

Symptomatic peripheral vascular disease affects 50% of diabetics at 20 years post-diagnosis and involves both large and small vessels. The large vessel involvement is due to accelerated atherosclerosis and the small vessels are involved as a result of structural and functional changes in the microvascular endothelium.

Infection is always a risk in poorly controlled and long-standing diabetes and this completes the picture seen in diabetic foot.

 The contributory factors leading to diabetic foot are: poor vision, decreased mobility in joints, cerebrovascular disease, peripheral oedema due to heart disease, autonomic denervation of sweat glands leading to dry and fissured skin, reduced plantar sensitivity, abnormal pressure areas.

Infection can start after trivial trauma as a result of tight ill-fitting footwear, during cutting of toe nails, callus formation or walking barefoot on an uneven hard surface.

- *Features of neuropathy*: foot deformities, neuropathic ulcers.
- *Features of ischaemia*: ulceration, colour changes, gangrene (usually wet).
- *Features of infection*: infection can be local and superficial or spreading cellulitis or an abscess or with associated osteomyelitis of the underlying bone.

The Charcot's joint was originally described in association with tabes dorsalis. This affects 0.2% of diabetics. Four factors are responsible for the onset of Charcot deformity:
- peripheral neuropathy
- autonomic neuropathy
- localised osteopenia
- trauma.

The acute phase is characterised by a red swollen and often painful foot which may last for several months.

 Thorough assessment of all the three underlying abnormalities:
- treatment of infection with appropriate antibiotics: amoxicillin plus metronidazole or augmentin (clindamycin and ciprofloxacin if allergic to penicillin)
- care of the ulcer if present: debridement, topical dressings
- tight diabetic control
- protection of the foot: total-contact casting which is minimally padded, moulded to the foot and allows for mobility while the ulcer heals
- treatment of underlying ischaemia.

**Other measures**
- The foot should be kept warm and moist to prevent formation of necrotic material, using various topical preparations such as alginates, hydrocolloids and foam. Hyperbaric oxygen is also used occasionally.
- Prevention of diabetic foot is more important and involves patient education and recognition of the foot at risk and early treatment.

**Your revision notes:**

## Carotid stenosis

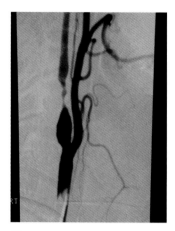

**Figure 3.14**

### Questions

**Q1** What investigation is this?

**Q2** What abnormality is demonstrated?

**Q3** What other imaging modalities can be used to demonstrate this abnormality?

**Q4** What is the typical presentation of these lesions when symptomatic?

**Q5** How would you manage a patient with symptoms related to this lesion?

## Answers

**(A1)** A digital subtraction carotid angiogram. Direct common carotid injection of contrast (catheter visible in picture).

**(A2)** A tight (95%) internal carotid artery stenosis.

**(A3)** Colour duplex sonography; MRA; CTA.

**(A4)**
- Carotid territory TIA or mini-stroke or PRIND (prolonged reversible ischaemic neurological deficit).
- Retinal emboli – amaurosis fugax.
- Recovered stroke.
- Sensory motor cortex distribution, hand, arm and face predominantly affected, speech disturbance in dominant cortex. Some higher cortical function disturbance in dominant hemisphere (dyspraxia etc).

**(A5)**
- Treat medical risk factors with antiplatelet therapy, statin, BP control.
- Assess fitness for carotid intervention.
- Consider for a carotid endarterectomy.
- Carotid stenting as part of a controlled trial in selected centres.

# Below-knee amputation (BKA)

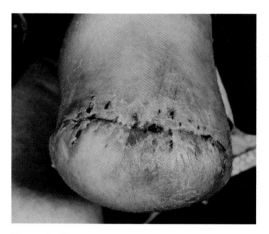

**Figure 3.15**

## Questions

**Q1** What operation has been performed on this patient?

**Q2** What are the indications for performing this operation?

**Q3** What complications would you have warned this patient of pre-operatively?

**Q4** What are the specific contra-indications to performing this operation?

**Q5** How would you pre-operatively assess and manage a patient undergoing this procedure?

## Answers

 Below-knee amputation: long posterior flap method.

- Complications of peripheral vascular disease (85%); diabetes (40%).
- Trauma (10%).
- Malignant tumours (3%), e.g. malignant melanoma.
- Infection.
- Congenital deformity.
- Chronic pain.
- 'Useless' limb: usually due to neurological injury.

 **Post-operative complications**
Remember early and late:
- early:
  - stump haematoma
  - flap necrosis, infection
  - stump trauma from falls
  - wound-related pain
- late:
  - neuroma formation
  - osteomyelitis
  - bony erosion
  - ulceration
  - ongoing ischaemia
  - phantom limb pain: good control with a combination of gabapentin and amitriptyline
  - joint contractures.

 **Specific contraindications to performing a BKA**
- Specific indication for performing a higher amputation.
- Fixed flexion deformity of knee.
- Inability to leave a tibial stump of at least 7.5 cm.
- Insufficient tissue for adequate healing.
- Bed-bound patients.

**Pre-operative work-up and assessment**
- Multidisciplinary approach in elective cases:
  - involve anaesthetic team (patient normally has a high ASA grade with multiple co-morbidities)
  - prosthetic specialist
  - nursing staff
  - physiotherapy
  - occupational therapist
  - psychologist.
- Obtain consent to amputate more proximally than intended.
- Assessment of level of amputation should include ability of patient to undergo successful rehabilitation:
  - energy expenditure with above-knee prosthesis > below knee prosthesis
  - may limit patients with co-existing IHD
  - above-knee amputation or through-knee amputation generally better for wheelchair-bound patient

- below-knee stump more liable to decubitus ulceration, therefore contraindicated in the bed-bound, also in those with a fixed flexion contracture >15 degrees.
- Level of amputation influenced by:
  - viability of tissues and degree of tissue loss
  - severity and pattern of vascular disease including consideration of previous vascular grafts
  - previous orthopaedic prostheses
  - underlying pathology (ensure pathology available)
  - functional requirement
  - comfort
  - cosmetic appearance
  - importance of preserving the knee joint and epiphysis in children.

**Assessment of blood supply**
- Most surgeons rely on clinical judgement.
- Unproven adjunctive tests include laser Doppler studies, transcutaneous measurement of oxygenation, measurement of blood flow in the skin using isotopes.
- Bony appraisal assessed by taking plain radiographs.

**Optimisation**
- Major amputation is high-risk surgery. Patients are normally ASA grade III/IV. Pre-operative preparation to minimise perioperative complications would include DVT prophylaxis and antibiotic prophylaxis.
- Urinary catheter to assess input/output and allow ease of micturition whilst bed-bound.

**Your revision notes:**

# Transmetatarsal amputation

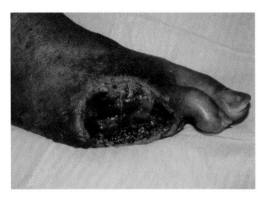

**Figure 3.16**

## Questions

**Q1** What type of amputation has been performed on this foot? What do you think was the initial indication?

**Q2** Where is the amputation made and why must the plantar skin be healthy?

**Q3** What is the complication of this operation seen here? What should be done?

**Q4** What types of amputation are there?

## Answers

 • Transmetatarsal amputation of the lateral three toes.
• Gangrene or infection affecting several toes.

 • Metatarsals divided at the mid-shaft level.
• Plantar skin must be healthy because the incision uses a total plantar flap.

 Wound infection and gangrene.
• Patient should be commenced on iv antibiotics after appropriate wound swabs taken for sensitivities.
• Plain radiograph to look for underlying osteomyelitis.
• Further debridement or higher amputation performed.

 **Types of amputation**
• Toe: most common. Usually through proximal phalanx. Must not be performed through the joint as that exposes avascular cartilage and it won't heal.
• Ray: excision of toe through the metatarsal bone.
• Transmetatarsal: divided at mid-shaft level. Indicated for infection or gangrene affecting several toes. Uses a *total* plantar flap. Provides excellent function post-operatively.
• Mid-foot: consider only in patients with correctable or absent ischaemia. Types include Lisfranc (disarticulation between metatarsal and tarsal bones) and Chopart (disarticulation of the talonavicular and calcaneocuboid joints). Main disadvantage unpredictable healing rates and development of equinus deformity, which limits ambulation.
• Ankle-level (Syme and Pirogoff): rarely indicated in vascular practice today.
• Below-knee (Burgess long posterior flap and skew flap): RCT comparing two showed same healing, revision and successful ambulation rates.
• Through-knee, e.g. Gritti–Stokes: useful if orthopaedic metalware in the femur precluded AKA. Unpredictable healing of skin flaps.
• Above-knee.
• Hip disarticulation and hindquarter:
  – malignant disease
  – extensive trauma
  – infection or gangrene
  – non-healing high AKA.

# Venous ulceration

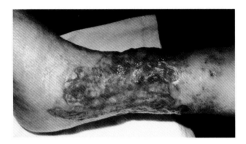

**Figure 3.17**

## Questions

**Q1** This picture shows an ulcer probably from what problem?

**Q2** What are the characteristic features of this type of ulcer?

**Q3** What points are important to obtain from the history and examination prior to treatment?

**Q4** What are the principles in management?

**Q5** What is the latest hypothesis postulated to explain venous ulceration?

## Answers

(A1) Likely to be due to venous insufficiency.

(A2) Longitudinal ulcer with sloping edges along the medial malleolus with a red granular base. Other signs that are seen are primarily due to venous disease:
- staining of the skin in gaiter area: thought to be due to blood leak from capillaries
- ankle flare: distension of tiny veins on the medial aspect of foot
- atrophy of skin
- lipodermatosclerosis
- evidence of any obvious varicose veins.

(A3) Ask for:
- previous history of deep vein thrombosis
- history of claudication pain to rule out arterial disease
- previous surgery for varicose veins or vein harvesting for CABG
- other medical conditions that can influence management.

Look for:
- ulcers and other stigmata of varicose veins and their distribution (great or the short system)
- foot pulses and ankle brachial pressure index
- site of any incompetence (SFJ/SPJ/other perforators).

(Learn to use Doppler to ascertain these prior to your clinical exam.)

(A4)
- A duplex scan is important to ascertain whether there is deep or superficial venous incompetence.
- If venous ulcer is due to superficial venous incompetence, treatment of varicose veins is recommended.
- If the ulcer is due to deep venous incompetence, dressing of ulcers and compression bandage (four-layer technique generating a pressure of up to 45 mmHg at ankle) is the recommended treatment. Beware of arterial disease before you embark on this line of management.

(A5) *'The white cell trapping hypothesis'*: venous hypertension causes increased sequestration of white cells in the microcirculation of the leg. These trapped leucocytes become activated and release oxygen free radicals and the proteolytic enzymes that are normally released in defence against infection. This in turn causes injury to capillary endothelium and leads to leg ulceration eventually.

# Ruptured abdominal aortic aneurysm

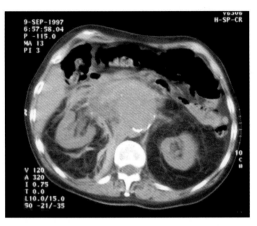

Figure 3.18

## Questions

Q1 What abnormality does this CT scan show?

Q2 How accurate is CT scanning for making this diagnosis?

Q3 Is intervention indicated for all patients?

Q4 What resuscitation is required?

Q5 Name six common complications after surgery for this condition.

## Answers

(A1) AAA with evidence of rupture (ill-defined outer margin on right side with blood tracking posteriorly on the right side).

(A2) 80–85% accuracy. False negatives are a concern in case the opportunity to repair the AAA is missed.

(A3) For most patients, but risk scores, e.g. Hardman index, do exist to predict poor survival in some patients who can be managed compassionately. Shock, history of loss of consciousness, anaemia, raised creatinine, and increasing age are poor prognostic indicators.

(A4) 'Permissive hypotension'. Do not aggressively treat shock with colloid because of the risk of further bleeding. Gain control by an aortic clamp or balloon as soon as possible in theatre, and then give fluids.

(A5)
- Coagulopathy.
- ATN/renal failure.
- Cardiac ischaemia/MI/cardiogenic shock.
- Peripheral thromboembolism.
- SIRS/MODS.
- Abdominal compartment syndrome.

# Carotid body tumour (chemodectoma)

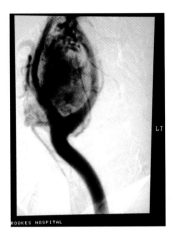

**Figure 3.19**

## Questions

(Q1) What investigation is this?

(Q2) What abnormality at the carotid bifurcation does it show?

(Q3) How do these lesions present?

(Q4) Why is a biopsy contraindicated?

(Q5) What other lesions are associated with this condition?

(Q6) How are these lesions managed?

## Answers

**(A1)** Digital subtraction angiogram (carotid).

**(A2)** A carotid body tumour, chemodectoma, with the classical tumour blush and splaying of the bifurcation.

**(A3)** Pulsatile neck lump.

**(A4)** High risk of excessive bleeding: these are highly vascular lesions.

**(A5)** Other paragangliomata, vagal, mediastinal, adrenal phaeochromocytomas. More common in bilateral carotid body tumours.

**(A6)**
- Excision, in view of low-grade malignant risk.
- Not radiosensitive but radiotherapy is occasionally used in elderly patients who are not suitable for surgery.
- Pre-operative embolisation to reduce vascularity is sometimes considered but there is no evidence that this is beneficial.
- Advanced tumours may require excision and grafting of the internal carotid artery.

# Lymphoedema

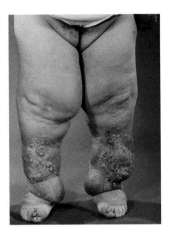

**Figure 3.20**

This 58-year-old lady has had this condition since birth.

## Questions

**Q1** Describe what you see. What is the most likely diagnosis?

**Q2** What are the differential diagnoses?

**Q3** What is the difference between primary and secondary lymphoedema?

**Q4** How would you investigate this problem?

**Q5** What are the treatment options available to this lady?

## Answers

- Gross bilateral leg swelling.
- Loss of contour at ankle: 'buffalo hump' over dorsum of foot.
- Skin looks thickened and indurated.
- **Milroy's disease**.

 Differential diagnoses of bilateral swollen legs:
- lymphoedema: primary and secondary
- central causes: right heart failure, hypoalbuminaemia, nephrotic syndrome and hypothyroidism
- peripheral or local causes: usually venous – deep vein thrombosis, chronic venous insufficiency, Klippel–Trénaunay syndrome
- rare causes: angio-oedema, arteriovenous malformations.

 **Primary lymphoedema**
- Refers to congenital disease or primary lymphatic failure: Milroy's disease.
- 3× more common in women.
- Underlying pathology originates within the lymphatics.

**Secondary lymphoedema**
Classification:
- malignancy: infiltration of the lymphatics
- infections, e.g. filiaris, tuberculosis
- post-surgery – axillary dissection in breast surgery or radiotherapy (inguinal irradiation).

- Exclude secondary causes.
- Use of lymphography and radionuclide lymphatic clearance studies.

 **Non-surgical (for over 90% cases)**
- Grade III compression stockings.
- Intermittent pneumatic compression device.
- Treat cellulitis aggressively.
- Advise patient to elevate limbs as much as possible and stress importance of hygiene and chiropody.
- Patient motivation is key.
- May take time to see improvement but can be very successful.

**Surgical**
- Used rarely and results generally poor.
- Lymph drainage procedures involve lympho-venous shunts or bridging operations.
- Debulking procedures to reduce volume of leg, e.g. Homans' procedure.

# Thoracoscopic sympathectomy

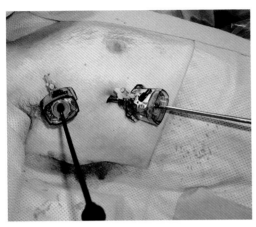

Figure 3.21

## Questions

Q1 This patient is undergoing a procedure to relieve excessive palmar sweating. What operation is this?

Q2 What are the complications of this procedure?

Q3 How does the operation work?

Q4 What are the features of Horner's syndrome?

Q5 Name three other causes of a Horner's syndrome.

## Answers

 Thoracoscopic T2 sympathectomy.

- Compensatory hyperhidrosis.
- Horner's syndrome.
- Pneumothorax.
- Haemothorax.
- Intercostal neuralgia.

 Removes the sympathetic stimulus for sweating from the thoracic sympathetic chain passing to the hand by division at the T2 level.

- Miosis.
- Partial ptosis.
- Anhydrosis.
- Enophthalmos.

- Syringomyelia.
- Pancoast's tumour.
- Carotid artery dissection.
- Neck trauma.
- Mid-brain/cervical spine tumour.

# Abdominal aortic aneurysm (AAA)

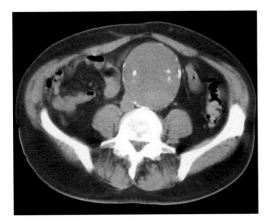

**Figure 3.22**

## Questions

**Q1** What is the definition of the condition depicted in the CT scan?

**Q2** How would you classify this condition?

**Q3** Where do they commonly occur and what do you know about their epidemiology?

**Q4** How do they present and what are their complications?

**Q5** What are the important factors in deciding when to operate electively on an abdominal aortic aneurysm and what investigations would you order pre-operatively?

## Answers

 Dilatation of part of an artery vessel or heart chamber by at least 100% (>50% = arteriomegaly or an ectatic artery).

 **Classification**
- *False*: due to a traumatic breach of the wall with the sac made up from the compressed surrounding tissue.
- *True*: dilatation involving all layers of the wall.
- *By shape*:
  - fusiform: spindle shaped involving whole of the circumference
  - saccular: small segment of wall ballooning due to localised weakness.
- *By cause*: acquired versus congenital
  - acquired: normally due to atherosclerosis
  - traumatic: popliteal artery aneurysms in horse-riders!
  - inflammatory: these rupture at a smaller diameter and can be very challenging at surgery
  - mycotic: infective, e.g. due to endocarditis. Syphilis – typically saccular and affecting the thoracic part of the aorta
  - connective tissue disorders: Marfan's, Ehlers–Danlos syndrome.

 • Commonest site is the abdominal aorta (2% finding at autopsy).
- Abdominal aortic aneurysms (AAA) are often associated with aneurysmal dilatation of the iliac, femoral and popliteal vessels.
- Popliteal aneurysms: most common peripheral aneurysm and second commonest overall.
- Splenic artery aneurysms: <1/10 000; 4 × greater in females especially during child-bearing years; 25% rupture, especially in third trimester.
- Intracranial 'berry' aneurysms: found at the junctions of the limbs to the circle of Willis. This is a congenital weakness.

**Epidemiology**
- Incidence: increases with age, 5% of over 50s; 15% of over 80s.
- Sex: M:F = 6:1.
- 12-fold risk for first-degree relatives affected.
- Distribution: aneurysms due to atherosclerosis found in abdominal aorta; 30% have iliac disease; 95% infrarenal.

 **Clinical features**
- Depend on site.
- 75% are asymptomatic: incidental finding during screening or investigation of other problems.
- Berry aneurysms: rupture causes subarachnoid haemorrhage.
- AAA: abdominal pain referred to the back (can be acute or chronic).

**Complications**
- Rupture.
- Thrombosis (causing lower limb ischaemia).
- Embolism.
- Fistulation: to bowel (aorto-enteric), to vena cava, renal vein.
- Pressure effects on adjacent organs.

**Management issues**
- Most important factor is size of the aneurysm:
  - repair all above 5.5 cm (UK Small Aneurysm Trial). Some surgeons would advocate repair at 6 cm in women because they are less prone to rupture
  - no benefit to repair at 4–5.5 cm: operative mortality outweighs risk of rupture. These patients should be enrolled on an annual USS screening programme and operated on when the aneurysm attains the requisite size.
- 5-year rupture rate 25% for >5 cm.
- Age limit for cut-off for surgery 85 years.
- Elective mortality: 1–5% in regional centres.
- Emergency: up to 80%.

**Investigations**
- CXR (thoracic extension).
- ECG.
- Echo: to aid in assessment of peri-operative risk.
- ESR: is there an inflammatory component?
- Urea and electrolytes: pre-operative renal failure is associated with a poorer prognosis.
- USS: size.
- CT: to look at juxtarenal anatomy. Need to avoid suprarenal clamping if at all possible. Also look at the distal extent of the aneurysm – directs need for a bifurcated graft if iliac arteries are involved.
- May require a 'stenting' CT if endovascular repair considered.

**Your revision notes:**

# Superior vena cava syndrome

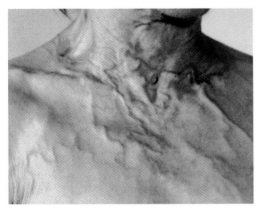

**Figure 3.23**

## Questions

**Q1** Describe the findings in the photograph. What is the diagnosis?

**Q2** What are the collaterals involved in the SVC compression?

**Q3** What are the causes?

**Q4** What are the symptoms in SVC compression?

**Q5** What are the signs in SVC compression?

**Q6** What are the diagnostic modalities available to evaluate the lesion?

**Q7** What is the management?

## Answers

 This is termed 'superior vena cava syndrome'. This is characterised by striking dilatation of the veins in the head and neck and the upper torso secondary to the obstruction of the SVC. There is bypassing of the obstruction and henceforth there is a dilatation of the other veins on the upper torso.

 An obstructed SVC initiates collateral venous return to the heart from the upper half of the body through four principal pathways:
- azygous venous system, which includes the azygous vein, the hemi-azygous vein, and the connecting intercostal veins
- the internal mammary venous system with its tributaries communicating to the superior and inferior epigastric veins
- the long thoracic venous system, with its connections to the femoral veins
- the vertebral plexus of veins.

If the level of obstruction is proximal to the azygous vein entry point into the SVC, then the effects are less drastic but if the obstruction is distal to the azygous entry then the effects are very severe.

 **Malignancy**
- Bronchogenic carcinoma (80%).
- Malignant lymphoma (15%).
- Metastatic disease (breast cancer, testicular seminoma, thyroid and thymic cancers, colon cancer).

**Benign disease (rare)**
- Mediastinal fibrosis
  - idiopathic
  - tuberculosis
  - histoplasmosis
  - actinomycosis.
- Vena cava thrombosis
  - idiopathic
  - long-term venous catheters, shunts or pacemakers
  - Behçet's syndrome
  - polycythaemia vera
  - paroxysmal nocturnal haemoglobinuria.
- Benign mediastinal tumour
  - aortic aneurysm
  - goitre
  - dermoid tumour
  - sarcoidosis.

- Dyspnoea (50%).
- Neck and facial swelling (40%).
- Swelling of the trunk and upper extremities (40%).
- Choking sensation.
- Cough.
- Stridor.
- Hoarseness of voice.
- Dysphagia.

- Chest pain.
- Head fullness or pressure sensation, headache.
- Lacrimation.

- Thoracic vein distention (65%).
- Neck vein distention (55%).
- Facial oedema (55%).
- Tachypnoea (40%).
- Plethora of the face and cyanosis (15%).
- Oedema of upper extremities (10%).
- Paralysis of the vocal cords (3%).
- Horner's syndrome (3%).
- Distended antecubital veins.

- Chest X-ray.
- MRI of the chest.
- CT scan of the chest.
- Doppler ultrasound.
- Radionuclide technetium Tc- 99m venography.
- Gallium PET scans.

1 Identify mass aetiology – controversial debates still exist between diagnosis first or treat first:
   – sputum cytology, bronchoscopy + biopsy, thoracoscopy, CT-guided biopsies, sternotomy or thoracotomy to obtain tissue for histology.
2 Supportive care: nursing the patient upright. Emergency treatment is indicated when brain oedema, decreased cardiac output, or upper airway oedema is present. Corticosteroids and diuretics are often used to relieve laryngeal or cerebral oedema:
   – ABC management
   – corticosteroids
   – diuretics.
3 Reduction in mass size – depending on the histology, either radiotherapy or chemotherapy depending on the best sensitivity profiles:
   – radiation therapy for radio-sensitive tumours (non-small-cell lung cancers)
   – chemotherapy (small-cell lung cancers, lymphomas).
4 Surgical decompression – commonly considered in benign cases and only rarely/isolated instances of malignancies:
   – surgical bypass
   – stenting.
5 Consider anticoagulation: especially if complicated by a luminal thrombus.

# Section 4

# Head and neck

## Osler–Weber–Rendu disease

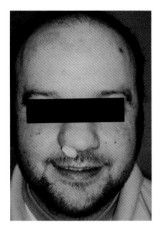

**Figure 4.1**

This 34-year-old male had multiple hospital admissions with recurrent epistaxis. There was a strong family history of epistaxis.

### Questions

Q1 What is the diagnosis?

Q2 What is the mode of inheritance?

Q3 How else may it present?

## Answers

 Osler–Weber–Rendu disease (hereditary haemorrhagic telangiectasia). Note the nasal pack and multiple telangiectasia on the skin of the face.

 Autosomal dominant.

 Haemoptysis, GI bleeding, genitourinary bleeding.

Osler–Weber–Rendu disease is an autosomal dominant disorder in which vessel walls lack contractile elements, and is characterised by multiple telangiectasia on skin and mucous membranes (*see* Figure 4.1). Troublesome epistaxis can be treated with repeated laser coagulation or skin grafting of the nasal cavity.

## Thyroglossal cyst

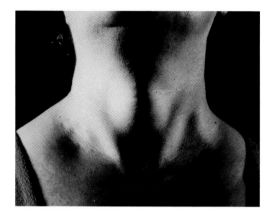

Figure 4.2

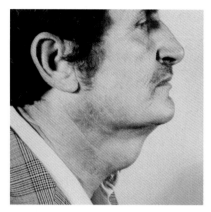

Figure 4.3

### Questions

(Q1) These two photographs (Figures 4.2 and 4.3) depict the same condition. What is your differential diagnosis?

(Q2) When this patient opens his mouth and sticks his tongue out, the swelling moves upwards. What is the diagnosis, and what do you understand by the condition?

(Q3) What do you know about the epidemiology of this condition?

(Q4) What is the embryological origin of this condition?

(Q5) What are the indications for surgery?

(Q6) How do you treat this condition? What are the possible complications?

(Q7) Can it turn malignant?

(Q8) The following photographs (Figures 4.4 and 4.5) show potential complications of this condition. What are they?

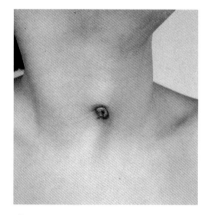

Figure 4.4

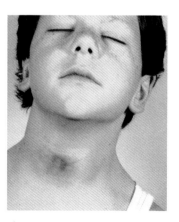

Figure 4.5

## Answers

**(A1)**
- Thyroglossal cyst.
- Thyroid nodules and masses (including a prominent pyramidal lobe).
- Enlarged lymph nodes.
- Dermoid/epidermoid cysts.
- Subhyoid bursae.

**(A2)** Thyroglossal cyst: this is a dilatation along the thyroglossal duct, the rest of which may or may not be obliterated.

**(A3)**
- Rare, worldwide distribution.
- M = F.
- Rarely present at birth, 40% present in the first decade of life. Can even present as late as the ninth decade. Generally appear between the ages of 15 and 30 years, more often in women.

**(A4)** Remnant from persistence of part of the thyroglossal tract, which marks the developmental descent of the thyroid gland. The thyroid appears as a midline diverticulum at the fourth week of gestation and descends ventrally from what will become the foramen caecum (posterior third of the tongue) down between the second branchial arches. The thyroglossal cyst is a portion of the thyroglossal duct, which remains patent.

- Thyroglossal cysts: 90% located in front of hyoid; 8% subhyoid; 2% lingual.

**(A5)**
- Cosmetic reasons.
- Discomfort.
- Risk of infection: these lumps are usually non-tender, but if they become infected or enlarged surgery may be needed.

**(A6)** Essentially surgical:
- Sistrunk's operation is operation of choice
- check first that this is not the only thyroid tissue in the patient, by performing a preliminary radio-iodine scan!
- make transverse incision over cyst, dissect cyst out, look for downward tract and excise it, then follow main tract upwards to hyoid bone. Excise middle third of hyoid bone and then excise rest of duct to its apex in continuity
- complications: haematoma, infection and recurrence (especially if central part of hyoid bone is not excised).

**(A7)** Yes. These cysts are lined by stratified squamous epithelium or ciliated pseudostratified epithelium. They may have lymphoid or thyroid tissue in wall. Can be site of ectopic thyroid, which may turn malignant – if so it is of the papillary type.

**(A8)**
- Figure 4.4: Thyroglossal sinus: acquired sinus following rupture or surgery for a thyroglossal cyst. From a surgical viewpoint this may be the result of not excising the tract completely.
- Note the crescenteric scaly midline nodule.

- Figure 4.5: Infection about to discharge onto the skin surface.

# Parotid tumour (1) and radiotherapy

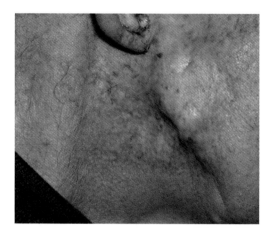

**Figure 4.6**

This 74-year-old male had a parotidectomy followed by radiotherapy for a malignant parotid tumour 40 years ago.

## Questions

Q1 What complications of radiotherapy are shown in this photograph?

Q2 Classify the complications of radiotherapy.

Q3 Give a basic classification of tumours of the parotid gland.

Q4 What clinical features are suggestive of malignancy?

Q5 What important complications should patients be warned of prior to parotidectomy?

Q6 What is Frey's syndrome?

## Answers

**A1** The most obvious complications in this case are thinning of the skin and the presence of telangiectasia.

**A2** Complications of radiotherapy are best thought of as early and late:
- early complications include bleeding, ulceration, mucositis, vomiting, diarrhoea and bone marrow suppression
- late complications include gonadal damage, damage to fine blood vessels (resulting in poor wound healing, tissue fibrosis, and telangiectasia), lymphoedema, and the induction of a second malignancy.

**A3**
- *Benign:*
  - pleomorphic adenoma
  - Warthin's tumour
  - oncocytoma.
- *Malignant:*
  - mucoepidermoid carcinoma
  - adenocarcinoma
  - acinic cell carcinoma
  - adenoid cystic carcinoma
  - squamous cell carcinoma.

**A4** It is often not possible to differentiate benign from malignant lesions clinically, but the presence of skin ulceration, a facial nerve palsy, pain, fixity, history of recent rapid growth and cervical lymphadenopathy are suggestive of malignancy.

**A5** Haematoma, salivary fistula, facial nerve palsy (temporary/permanent), Frey's syndrome.

**A6** Salivation is under parasympathetic autonomic control. In Frey's syndrome the parasympathetic branches that have been sectioned intra-operatively form aberrant connections with the local skin sweat glands, resulting in gustatory sweating (sweating and flushing of the overlying skin during eating, or even in anticipation of food).

# Lymphadenopathy

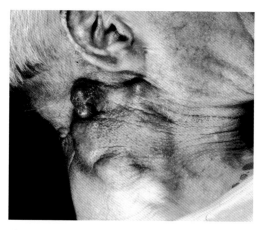

**Figure 4.7**

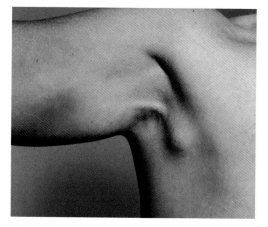

**Figure 4.8**

## Questions

Q1 What do Figures 4.7 and 4.8 show?

Q2 How do you classify cervical lymph nodes anatomically?

Q3 What are the causes of cervical lymphadenopathy?

Q4 How would you further investigate this patient?

## Answers

 • Figure 4.7: cervical lymphadenopathy + likely metastases from a head or neck tumour.
• Figure 4.8: axillary lymphadenopathy.

 • Superficial and deep cervical.
• Supraclavicular.
• Submandibular.
• Parotid.
• Submental.
• Pre- and post-auricular.

 • *Generalised*:
 – lymphoma or leukaemia
 – infections: HIV, EBV, TB
 – infiltration: sarcoid.
• *Localised*:
 – spread from malignant head and neck tumours (melanoma, nasopharyngeal carcinoma, thyroid carcinoma)
 – head and neck infection.

 • Full history and examination including other nodes, full ENT examination, liver, spleen etc.
• CXR (sarcoid, TB, mediastinal lymphadenopathy from haematological malignancies).
• Lymph node excision biopsy or FNA.
• CT of the chest and abdomen if indicated (for diagnosis and staging).

# Cystic hygroma

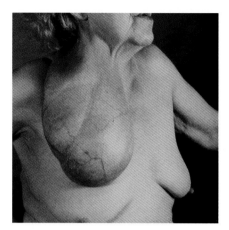

**Figure 4.9**

### Questions

**Q1** What is the diagnosis?

**Q2** What is its pathology?

**Q3** What symptoms may the patient be experiencing?

**Q4** If you were unsure of the diagnosis, what investigations could you perform to aid you?

**Q5** How would you treat the condition?

This 70-year-old lady presented to clinic with this abnormality, which has been present since birth. It has gradually got larger and is now causing her to have symptoms. On examination it is a soft, fluctuant lobulated cystic swelling that seems to originate from the posterior triangle of the neck. It is brilliantly transilluminable.

## Answers

(A1) A cystic hygroma.

(A2) A cystic hygroma is a congenital lymphatic malformation lying at the root of the neck. It consists of thin-walled interconnecting cysts formed from the coalescence of the early lymphatic elements during development. This is found in the posterior triangle of the neck. Most are present from birth (40–65%), but some can develop late.

(A3) • Obstruction of respiratory organs: therefore difficulty in breathing.
• Obstruction of swallowing.
• Cosmetic problems.

(A4) Mainly radiological:
• CXR: to map the caudal extent of the cystic hygroma.
• CT/MRI especially if complex.

(A5) • Non-surgical: aspiration and injection of sclerosant (generally unsuccessful).
• Surgical: may be partial to relieve symptoms or complete (as a one-stage procedure).

## Carcinoma of the tongue

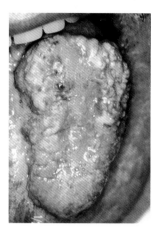

**Figure 4.10**

### Questions

(Q1) Describe what you see in this photograph.

(Q2) What is the diagnosis?

(Q3) What are the risk factors for developing this condition?

(Q4) Where are the most common sites of involvement?

(Q5) How do you think the patient presented?

(Q6) What is the treatment?

## Answers

 Photograph of a tongue.
- Tongue is deviated to the patient's left.
- Gross appearance shows an ulcerated lateral border with a rolled edge extending to the posterior third. Typical of an epithelioma.

 Carcinoma of the tongue.

 The six Ss: smoking, spicy food, syphilis, spirits, sepsis (poor oral hygiene), sharp tooth.

Leukoplakia, which appears as a white plaque that cannot be rubbed off, is an important pre-malignant condition and 14–18% of these eventually progress to form invasive carcinoma. Erythroplakia, a red mucosal plaque, is even more dangerous in terms of malignant transformation.

 • Anterior two-thirds of the tongue (75%) versus posterior one-third (25%).
- Most common on lateral borders (85%) from which the tumour extends directly to involve the floor of the mouth.

 **Symptoms**
- The common presenting symptoms consist of halitosis after ulceration has occurred, difficulty in swallowing, especially when the tumour has spread to the floor of the mouth due to fixation of the tongue and local rigidity.
- Local pain.
- Visible or palpable lesion on the tongue.
- Possible enlargement of cervical nodes.
- May present with otalgia: referred pain from cranial nerves V, IX, X.

**Signs**
- Deviation of tongue to the side of lesion (classical): due to fixation of tongue to underlying tissues by infiltration.
- Areas of leukoplakia.
- Enlarged lymph nodes: presence related to the size of the tumour. Metastases to regional lymph nodes present in 60% of patients when the tumour is over 2 cm in diameter.

 • Confirm diagnosis with biopsy first.
- With management of tumours in the aerodigestive tract: radiotherapy then salvage surgery.
- Underlying histology is a squamous cell carcinoma therefore sensitive to radiotherapy. Remove any teeth that may be in the field of radiation, to avoid the possibility of osteoradionecrosis of the mandible.
- Limited cervical block dissection may be required if enlarged cervical nodes do not resolve.
- *Stages 1 and 2*: both radiotherapy and surgery produce similar results.
- *Stages 3 and 4*: surgery followed by radiotherapy will have better results. Advanced cancers will require reconstruction after resection. The primary tumour can be resected by a transoral hemiglossectomy or partial glossectomy. Total glossectomy or glossolaryngectomy may sometimes be required. The floor of the mouth or mandible will also require to be removed en-bloc if involved. Elective lymph node dissection is suggested in view of the high incidence of nodal recurrence.

## Acute lymphadenitis

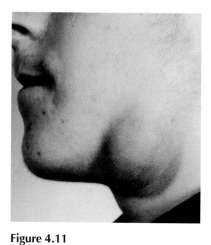

**Figure 4.11**

This young immigrant presented with this painful hot tender lump in his neck.

## Questions

**Q1** What is your clinical diagnosis?

**Q2** If this was a relatively painless abscess and the skin overlying it showed no evidence of increased heat or erythema, i.e. a 'cold' abscess, what would be the diagnosis?

**Q3** In what racial groups would you consider this possibility?

**Q4** At operation, the infected lymph node had broken down through the deep fascia and the abscess lay in the subcutaneous tissues. What is this type of abscess called?

**Q5** What would happen if the abscess were left untreated?

## Answers

(A1) Acute lymphadenitis.

(A2) Tuberculous cervical adenitis with an overlying abscess.

(A3) Immigrants from Third World countries where tuberculosis is still common.

(A4) A collar abscess.

(A5) The abscess will discharge onto the skin and result in a chronic tuberculous sinus.

# Parotid tumour (2)

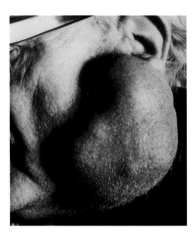

**Figure 4.12**

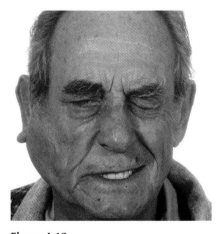

**Figure 4.13**

## Questions

**Q1** What is the differential diagnosis and what is the most likely diagnosis?

**Q2** What are the commonest tumours in this area?

**Q3** How can you distinguish clinically between whether this is a benign or malignant lesion?

**Q4** How may the diagnosis be confirmed? And how would you manage this swelling?

**Q5** What are the specific complications of a parotidectomy?

**Q6** Look at Figure 4.13. Describe what you see. What is the most likely diagnosis?

A 49-year-old gentleman presented to the outpatients with this slow-growing, painless swelling over his left mandible (Figure 4.12).

# Answers

 Divide lesions into those arising inside and outside the parotid gland.

**Arising inside the parotid gland**
- Neoplasia
  - benign: pleomorphic adenoma
  - malignant
  - lymphoma and leukaemia.*
- Stones.
- Infection and inflammation
  - mumps*
  - acute sialadenitis
  - HIV
  - salivary gland disease.
- Autoimmune: Sjögren's syndrome.*
- Infiltration: sarcoidosis.*
- Parotid lymph node enlargement.
- Neural origin: facial nerve neuroma.
- Vascular origin: temporal artery aneurysm.
- Systemic diseases
  - alcoholic liver disease
  - diabetes mellitus
  - pancreatitis
  - acromegaly
  - malnutrition.

**Arising outside the parotid gland**
- Soft tissue, e.g. lipoma or sebaceous cyst.
- Dental origin: infection.
- Muscular origin: masseter muscle hypertrophy.
- Bony origin: winged mandible.
- Neoplasia: infratemporal fossa and parapharyngeal tumours.

*Can present as bilateral swellings.

The most likely diagnosis is a pleomorphic adenoma.

- 90% of parotid gland tumours arise from salivary tissue, 90% of adenomas are benign, 90% of which lie in the superficial lobe.
- 75% are pleomorphic in nature.

**Pleomorphic adenoma**
- Most common parotid tumour
  - firm with a well-defined border
  - have an irregular surface
  - these require careful excision as local recurrence is common if incompletely excised
  - there is a small risk of malignant transformation.
- Occurs normally <50 years old.
- Facial nerve involvement rare.
- Found in tail of parotid, superficial to upper part of sternocleidomastoid.

**Adenolymphoma (Warthin's tumour)**
- Softer more mobile and slower growing.

- Occur >50 years old.
- Smoking important risk factor.
- Facial nerve rarely involved.
- Found in tail of parotid, superficial to upper part of sternocleidomastoid.
- Normally easier to remove.
- Does not recur locally.
- Rarely undergoes malignant transformation.

**Neoplasms of intermediate malignancy**
- Acinar cell and mucoepidermoid.

**Malignant tumours**
- Adenocarcinoma and adenocystic carcinoma.

Non-salivary tumours include lymphoma.

(A3) Clinical features that would make you suspicious that this lesion is malignant include:
- rapid growth and pain: localised or referred otalgia
- hyperaemic hot skin
- hard consistency
- fixed to skin and underlying muscle
- irregular surface or ill-defined edge
- facial nerve involvement
- lingual nerve infiltration in malignant tumours of the submandibular gland producing numbness of the anterior two-thirds of the tongue.

(A4) 
- A fine needle aspiration will confirm the diagnosis without risk of seeding the tumour.
- MRI can exclude deep lobe involvement.
- Surgical treatment is superficial parotidectomy (if only the superficial lobe is involved). While removing the tumour, avoid disrupting the capsule, otherwise local recurrence is high.
- Total parotidectomy with preservation of the facial nerve if both lobes or the deep lobe are involved.

(A5) Always divide into:
- immediate:
  - facial nerve transection
  - reactionary haemorrhage
- early:
  - wound infection
  - neuropraxia affecting facial nerve
  - salivary fistula
  - division of the greater auricular nerve: loss of sensation to the pinna of the ear
- late:
  - wound dimple
  - Frey's syndrome (see Parotid tumour (1) answer 6, p. 174 for details).

(A6) This patient has a swelling over his mandible. He is demonstrating weakness of his facial nerve (right side) on attempting to shut his eyes. The most probable diagnosis is a malignant tumour affecting his right parotid gland.

**Your revision notes:**

# Multinodular goitre

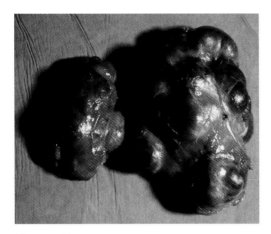

Figure 4.14

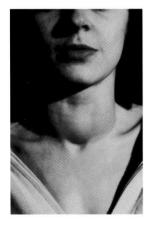

Figure 4.15

## Questions

**Q1** Describe what you see in Figure 4.14. What is the underlying diagnosis, bearing in mind the specimen is taken from the lady in Figure 4.15?

**Q2** What is the pathophysiology of this condition?

**Q3** What are the features of this condition?

**Q4** How may a patient with this present?

**Q5** When would you investigate a patient presenting with this problem, and what investigations would you institute and why?

**Q6** What are the indications for surgery in this condition?

**Q7** If this condition became toxic, how would you differentiate it from Graves' disease?

## Answers

**A1**
- Gross examination of the thyroid shows it consists of two separate thyroid masses, one being larger than the other. Both masses are multinodular with nodules of varying size and shape. The smaller is slightly more uniform with these distinct nodules also visible on the smaller specimen. The overall features of both pieces of tissue are those of a multinodular goitre. This is a diffuse process. However, certain nodules may be more prominent than others, and some nodules may present as a prominent nodule, even though this is part of a multinodular process.
- Figure 4.15 shows a young lady with a nodular swelling in her neck: likely goitre.

**A2** Multinodular goitre (MNG) results from disordered thyroid metabolism where some areas of the gland become hyperplastic and form nodules that later degenerate, fibrose, or calcify. MNG may arise primarily or develop from a pre-existing smooth enlargement.

**A3**
- Progression of a simple diffuse goitre to nodular enlargement.
- Middle-aged women.
- Positive family history.
- Malignant change occurs in 5% of untreated MNGs.
- Mild hyperthyroidism in overactive parts of gland (Plummer's syndrome).
- There are no eye signs (cf Graves' disease).

**A4**
- Cosmetic reasons/noticed lump in neck.
- Discomfort.
- Dyspnoea: tracheal compression.
- Dysphagia: oesophageal compression.
- Onset of hyperthyroidism.
- Worries about malignancy.

**A5** Investigate if prominent nodule present and features suggestive of malignancy such as cervical lymphadenopathy or recurrent laryngeal nerve palsy. Investigate with:
- TFTs (thyroid status).
- USS: gives the dimensions of goitre and nodules, look for cysts, which can be aspirated.
- CXR: retrosternal component?
- Nuclear medicine scan: hot and cold nodules.
- FNA (cold nodules).

**A6**
- Obstructive symptoms.
- Suspicion of malignancy.
- Thyrotoxicosis.
- Retrosternal extension.
- Increasing size despite adequate thyroxine therapy.
- Cosmesis.

**A7** Ways of differentiating between toxic MNG and Graves' disease are given in Table 4.1.

**Table 4.1** Characteristics of MNG and Graves' disease

| Toxic MNG | Graves' disease |
| --- | --- |
| Older | Younger |
| Nodular enlargement | Diffuse enlargement |
| No eye signs | Eye signs present |
| AF common in 40% of patients | AF uncommon |
| No associated autoimmune diseases | Association with other autoimmune problems |

## Sialadenitis

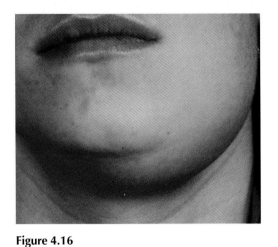

**Figure 4.16**

### Questions

**Q1** What is the diagnosis and origin of the swelling?

**Q2** What are the usual presenting symptoms?

**Q3** What is the aetiology of this problem?

**Q4** How is this condition investigated?

**Q5** What are the treatment options?

A 22-year-old lady presented with recurrent episodes of pain and the above swelling.

## Answers

 Recurrent sialadenitis in the submandibular gland.

- Painful swelling during eating or drinking (post-prandial).
- They are characterised by repeated episodes of pain and inflammation, usually leading to parenchymal degeneration and fibrous replacement of the gland substance. Predisposition to repeated episodes of secondary infection may be attributed to duct obstruction or to duct dilatation and depressed glandular secretion.
- Patient may have symptom-free intervals of a few weeks to several months.

 The pathogenesis is primarily stasis of salivary secretions secondary to obstruction or decreased salivary secretions.
- *Obstructive*:
  - stricture
  - sialolith
  - sialectasia
  - mucus plug
  - extrinsic ductal compression.
- *Non-obstructive*:
  - Sjögren's syndrome
  - sarcoidosis
  - lymphoma.

Salivary calculi are most commonly discovered in association with chronic sialadenitis, and their development is responsible for the recurrent nature of this disease; 80% of salivary duct stones develop in the submandibular duct, with 19% in the parotid and the remaining 1% in the sublingual gland. The factors favouring stones in the submandibular gland/duct are the mucoid nature of secretion and the flow against gravity.

Development of a submandibular salivary duct stone is the primary process that results in impaired salivary flow and ductal inflammation, which secondarily encourages retrograde bacterial migration and resultant sialadenitis.

- Plain X-ray: a radio-opaque calculus can usually be seen.
- Contrast sialogram: useful in radiolucent stones and also to demonstrate ductal ectasia and sialectasis.
- CT.

Salivary calculi are composed of calcium phosphate and carbonate, combined with magnesium, zinc and ammonium salts and organic material (cellular debris).

- The acute episode is treated with adequate hydration, gland massage, local heat, sialagogues and antibiotics (if there is evidence of infection).
- Stones that are palpable near the ductal orifice can be moved manually towards the orifice and removed. The orifice can be enlarged (incision) to extrude the stone. An incision can be made on the duct directly over the stone in order to remove it. Marsupalisation of the duct to the surrounding mucosa is then carried out.
- Sialodochoplasty has been tried for stricture with not much success.
- Excision of the gland can be undertaken in cases where conservative management has failed.
- Other modes of treatment tried are low-dose irradiation, tympanic neurectomy and ductal ligation, which have proven ineffective. Recently extracorporeal shock wave lithotripsy has been used in salivary duct stones.

## Thyroid carcinoma

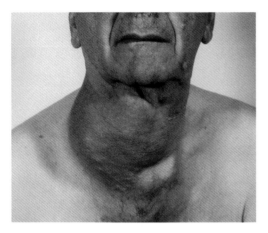

**Figure 4.17**

A 71-year-old male presented with this lump of 2 months' duration associated with hoarseness of voice.

## Questions

(Q1) What is the diagnosis?

(Q2) Describe the types and aetiology. Which type does this gentleman probably have and why?

(Q3) How do you investigate this lesion?

(Q4) Name a staging system for this tumour.

(Q5) What are the treatment options?

## Answers

 Carcinoma in the thyroid gland.
- It is an uncommon condition and it constitutes 1% of all malignancies. It is the commonest endocrine tumour. Incidence is 1–2 in 100 000. It is more common in females.
- The typical symptom is a fast-growing lesion in the thyroid region. It can be a solitary nodule or multinodular. Patients may present with symptoms of hoarseness of voice and difficulty in swallowing and breathing.
- Suspicious features of malignant thyroid lesions are short history, rapid increase in size, hoarseness of voice.
- Clinically (typically examined standing behind the patient) there is a firm, fixed and irregular lump which is moving with deglutition, with cervical and supraclavicular lymphadenopathy.
- In advanced cases the patient might have stridor or haemoptysis.
- Concomitant thyrotoxicosis makes malignancy less likely but does not exclude it.

 Pathologically they are classified as:
- well differentiated
  - papillary
  - follicular
  - mixed follicular–papillary
- Hürthle cell variant
- anaplastic (undifferentiated)
- medullary
- lymphoma
- others: secondaries.

### Aetiology
- In most the aetiology is not evident.
- Ionising radiation: papillary carcinoma.
- Low dietary iodine intake: follicular carcinoma.
- Familial: medullary.
- *Papillary carcinoma* is the commonest (72%) variant. It is commoner in young adults and children. It is commoner in iodine-rich areas and following exposure to ionising radiation. It spreads by a lymphatic route. Blood spread is a late feature. It presents as a solitary nodule and occasionally presents as cervical lymphadenopathy (lateral aberrant thyroid). It is multifocal, unencapsulated and involves lymph nodes.
- *Follicular carcinoma* (12%) is commoner in areas of low dietary iodine intake. The mean age of occurrence is 50 years. They present as a solitary nodule. Unlike papillary carcinoma, FNAC is usually unhelpful because it is difficult to differentiate between a follicular carcinoma and an adenoma. The final diagnosis usually rests on histological examination following resection. It tends to spread by the bloodstream. Distant metastases occur in the lungs and bone. Lymphatic feature is a late feature. It occurs as solitary and encapsulated forms.
- *Anaplastic tumour* is rare (5%) and commonly occurs in the elderly. It has a higher incidence in areas of endemic goitre. It has a very poor prognosis as it is a rapidly growing tumour which infiltrates the local surrounding tissue and metastasises into the bloodstream and lymphatics early. It is usually fixed, causing dyspnoea, stridor, hoarseness and dysphagia at presentation.

- *Medullary carcinoma* is a rare tumour that occurs in the parafollicular C cells of the thyroid. It is a solid tumour, which is unilateral in sporadic cases and usually bilateral in familial cases. It can be accompanied by diarrhoea caused by hormones. They are slow-growing tumours; however they metastasise via the bloodstream and lymphatics. Blood calcitonin levels can be a useful tumour marker, especially for recurrence after surgery.

This gentleman probably has an anaplastic tumour: see explanation above.

- Clinical examination.
- ENT examination: vocal cords examination is mandatory.
- Thyroid function.
- Calcium and autoantibody status.
- FNAC: for diagnosis.
- Plasma calcitonin: if medullary carcinoma is suspected.
- CXR.
- In large and fixed tumours a CT/MRI scan is done to exclude retrosternal extension.
- A solitary nodule may be investigated with iodine 123 or technetium 99 scintiscanning. Isotopically cold nodules that are solid and partly cystic are regarded as suspicious of malignancy.

American Joint Committee on cancer classification system for well-differentiated thyroid cancer.

**TNM staging**
- Primary tumour (T):
  - T1: $\leq 2$ cm intrathyroidal
  - T2: >2 cm and <4 cm intrathyroidal
  - T3: >4 cm intrathyroidal or any tumour with minimal extrathyroid extension
  - T4a: extends outside thyroid capsule and invades any of the following: subcutaneous tissue, larynx, trachea, oesophagus, recurrent laryngeal nerve
  - T4b: tumour invades the paravertebral fascia or mediastinal vessels or encases carotid artery.

All anaplastic/undifferentiated carcinomas are considered T4.

- Regional lymph nodes (N):
  - Nx: regional lymph nodes can be assessed
  - N0: no regional lymph node metastasis
  - N1: regional lymph node metastasis
  - N1a: metastasis in pre-tracheal or paratracheal nodes
  - N1b: metastasis in other unilateral, bilateral or contralateral cervical or mediastinal lymph nodes.

- Distant metastasis(M):
  - Mx: distant metastasis cannot be assessed
  - M0: no distant metastasis
  - M1: distant metastasis.

- Papillary carcinoma:
  - intrathyroid: hemithyroidectomy + thyroxine
  - extrathyroid: total thyroidectomy + modified block dissection of the neck + thyroxine + $^{131}$I (radio-iodine therapy).

- Follicular carcinoma:
  - total thyroidectomy + $^{131}$I + thyroxine.
- Medullary carcinoma:
  - total thyroidectomy + block dissection of neck
  - calcitonin assays: follow-up.
- Anaplastic:
  - resection, if possible, usually debulking
  - radiotherapy, usually palliative.
- Lymphoma:
  - radiotherapy is the first choice as these tumours are very radiosensitive
  - thyroidectomy, occasionally (or biopsy)
  - chemotherapy, rarely.

## Branchial cyst

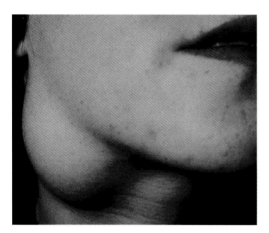

**Figure 4.18**

This 30-year-old adult presented with a slowly enlarging painless, cystic swelling in the neck.

## Questions

**Q1** What is the likely diagnosis? What is the differential diagnosis?

**Q2** Is this cystic swelling likely to be transilluminant and why?

**Q3** What is the embryological basis or development of this structure?

**Q4** How would you make a diagnosis of this mass and what investigation may be helpful?

**Q5** What complication may it undergo?

**Q6** How would you treat it?

## Answers

(A1) • Branchial cyst.
• Differential: TB abscess.

(A2) No: opaque on transillumination, due to desquamated epithelial cell contents.

(A3) • The second branchial arch in the fetus grows down over the third and fourth arches to form the cervical sinus. This usually disappears but its persistence is believed to lead to the formation of a branchial cyst, sinus or fistula.
• An alternative hypothesis is an acquired condition due to cystic degeneration in cervical lymphatic tissue. The cysts are lined by squamous epithelium.

(A4) History and clinical examination:
• usually presents in a young adult in the third decade
• M = F
• anterior triangle of neck in front of the upper third of the sternocleidomastoid
• smooth firm swelling that is ovoid in shape
• fluctuant on palpation
• look carefully for the opening of a fistula in this area
• FNA: opalescent fluid containing cholesterol crystals or pus.

(A5) • Infection: may then become hard and fixed to surrounding structures.
• Branchial sinus formation and discharge.

(A6) • Surgical excision of the cyst. This may be difficult if infected.
• Bonney's blue dye can be injected into the fistula/sinus allowing accurate surgical excision and therefore reducing recurrence rates.
• Complicating infections: treat with antibiotics.

# Section 5

# Neurosurgery

# Acute subdural haematoma

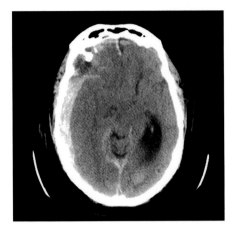

**Figure 5.1**

This 36-year-old man was involved in a road traffic accident. His GCS was 13 at the scene (E3V4M6). After admission to A&E, his GCS dropped to 7/15 (E0V2M5). He underwent a CT scan of his head.

## Questions

**Q1** What is the diagnosis?

**Q2** What is the immediate management of this patient?

**Q3** The patient's right pupil becomes abnormally dilated during transfer; what has happened?

**Q4** What manoeuvres or interventions could be performed in the ambulance?

**Q5** Why does the pupil dilate often before any motor effects on the IIIrd nerve?

**Q6** What definitive procedure does this patient require when he reaches the neurosurgical centre?

## Answers

(A1) Acute subdural haematoma.

(A2) ABC + immediate referral to the neurosurgical registrar on-call.

(A3) Raised intracranial pressure has probably resulted in IIIrd cranial nerve palsy as the uncus on the right has trapped the IIIrd nerve against the free edge of the tentorium. This is a heralding sign of full tentorial herniation.

(A4)
- Mannitol bolus (20%) or hypertonic saline. Possibly load with phenytoin/use of benzodiazepines to control seizures. Head up 30 degrees (taking care to immobilise cervical spine).
- An accompanying anaesthetist may wish to try mild hyperventilation to keep the $P_{CO_2}$ around 4.5 kPa.

(A5) The parasympathetic fibres supplying sphincter pupillae are found on the *outside* of the IIIrd nerve and are therefore the first to get damaged.

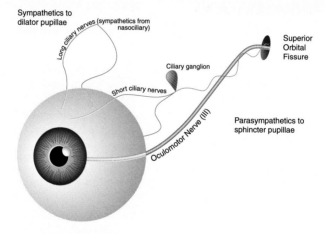

(A6) Craniotomy and evacuation of haematoma +/– postoperative ICP monitoring.

## Brain abscess

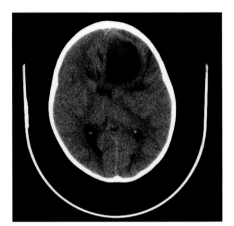

**Figure 5.2**

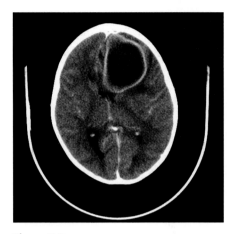

**Figure 5.3**

A 64-year-old woman with a prosthetic heart valve presents with a one-week history of a febrile illness. While being investigated for this, she develops a unilateral facial weakness and slurred speech. A CT scan with contrast was performed (pre-contrast on left, post-contrast on right).

## Questions

(Q1) What is the differential diagnosis of this CT scan given the history?

(Q2) What should be the management of this patient?

## Answers

 • Abscess.
• Intrinsic primary brain tumour.
• Intrinsic secondary tumour (metastasis).

 Given that this is a likely abscess, the management needs to be split into two.
1 Full investigation for the source of the sepsis:
   – repeated blood cultures
   – transthoracic echo (TTE) +/– transoesophageal echo (TOE) (given prosthetic heart valve)
   – CXR.

2 Diagnosis and treatment of the cerebral lesion:
   – stereotactic biopsy and aspiration followed by cytology and culture: this procedure will inform further management, e.g. antibiotics +/– oncology.

# Acute extradural haematoma

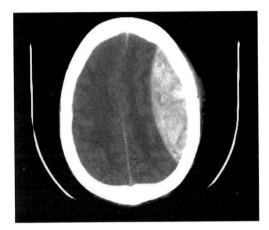

**Figure 5.4**

A 45-year-old man is on the golf course and he is unfortunately struck in the side of the head by an errant ball. Following his subsequent lacklustre performance on the back nine, he retires to the clubhouse where he complains to his friends that he has a headache. Several gin and tonics later, slurring his words and somewhat confused, he tells his friends that he is going to lie down. Half an hour following this, his friends find him unresponsive.

On admission to A&E, his GCS is 6 (E0V2M4) and he is therefore intubated and ventilated. A CT of his head is shown in Figure 5.4.

## Questions

Q1  What is the diagnosis?

Q2  What should be your immediate management of this patient?

Q3  Explain the anatomy behind this pathology.

Q4  Why is this pathology more localised than a subdural haematoma?

Q5  If, for some reason, transfer is delayed, what measures could you institute in discussion with neurosurgery?

## Answers

**A1** It shows a left extradural haematoma (EDH) with midline shift. There is also a small subgaleal haematoma on the left. This is the classic appearance of an EDH: a high density biconvex lesion adjacent to the skull.

**A2** *Always* A,B,C and then D(isability). So following stabilisation of the patient and securing the airway, he needs urgent referral to the on-call neurosurgical registrar with a view to urgent craniotomy and evacuation of the haematoma.

**A3** In contrast to the subdural haematoma, the extradural is the result of an arterial bleed and is in the space above the meninges. There is usually little direct brain damage and the haematoma exerts its effect by direct mass effect, so giving the classical clinical picture of a lucent period before deterioration. In this case, the likely artery to have been disrupted is the anterior branch of the middle meningeal artery as it courses past a pterional fracture.

**A4** An extradural haematoma strips the dura from the skull but respects the skull sutures as the dura is very tightly adherent to these. In contrast, a subdural haematoma, being below this layer, will not respect the anatomical landmarks of the skull sutures, and is thus thinner and more spread out (classically concave rather than convex).

**A5** Medical measures to control ICP:
- mannitol 20% iv bolus
- hypertonic saline
- head up 30 degrees (taking care of cervical spine if not cleared)
- phenytoin/benzodiazepines for control of seizures.

# Brain metastasis

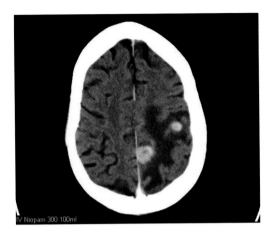

IV Niopam 300 100ml

**Figure 5.5**

A 62-year-old man is admitted to A&E via the GP with a progressive hemiplegia and slurred speech. He is afebrile. A diagnosis of stroke is made. A few days following admission, a CT is finally performed. Results are shown in Figure 5.5 (post-contrast).

## Questions

**Q1** What is the differential diagnosis of this CT scan given the history?

**Q2** What investigations should be undertaken?

**Q3** On further questioning and examination, it turns out that he had had a left lobectomy 12 months previously for non-small-cell lung cancer but he had been declared 'in remission'. What is the likely diagnosis? Give an outline of the management.

## Answers

 • Secondary intrinsic tumour (metastasis).
• Primary brain tumour.
• Cerebral abscess.

 • Bloods: including CRP, WCC (to attempt to rule out abscess).
• CXR/chest CT to rule out lung malignancy and sepsis.
• +/– abdomen/pelvis CT/liver USS.
• +/– endoscopy depending on history (anything to suggest colonic malignancy?).

 The most likely diagnosis is a brain metastasis secondary to his original lung primary. Since the slurred speech and hemiplegia may be a result of cortical oedema rather than direct invasion at this stage, a trial of steroids should be instituted. Secondly, the disease should be restaged with repeat CTs. An MRI of the head should be performed to look for smaller brain metastases. If this proves to be a solitary lesion in an otherwise healthy patient without other distant disease and if the lesion was superficial and in a non-eloquent area, craniotomy and excision could be considered. He will obviously require referral to the oncologists no matter what the decision regarding surgery.

## Carotid atheroma

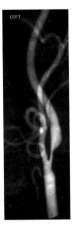

**Figure 5.6**

A 75-year-old man presents to your outpatients clinic having been referred by the GP. Last week he was having dinner with his wife when suddenly he was unable to use the right side of his body and suffered severely slurred speech. These symptoms resolved within a few hours. When the GP examined him his peripheral neurological examination was entirely normal and the only positive finding was bilateral carotid bruits.

## Questions

**Q1** Which arterial territory is consistent with this type of transient ischaemic attack?

**Q2** What should be the next investigations?

**Q3** Following first-line investigations, an angiogram is performed and is shown in Figure 5.6. What is the diagnosis?

**Q4** What would you recommend to the patient should be the next course of action?

**Q5** What are the complications associated with the surgical procedure most commonly used to address this pathology?

**Q6** What intraoperative monitoring can be used when this operation is performed under general anaesthetic, to reduce the possibility of specific complications?

**Q7** Are there any trials supporting your advice to the patient?

## Answers

(A1) Left carotid artery territory.

(A2) Carotid duplex in the first instance often followed by angiography of some description (either conventional X-ray angiography, MRA or CTA).

(A3) >75% stenosis of the left ICA.

(A4) Intervention: either carotid endarterectomy under LA or GA/or endovascular stenting of the left ICA.

(A5) Carotid endarterectomy: complications general and specific as always. Specific include approx 3% or less risk of death or neurological accident, 5% risk of cranial nerve palsy (either hypoglossal or cervical plexus), 1% or less risk of hyperperfusion syndrome.

(A6) Transcranial Doppler monitoring of the middle cerebral artery to detect embolic showers as a result of manipulation of the carotid arteries.

(A7) For symptomatic carotid disease, the North American Symptomatic Carotid Endarterectomy Trial (NASCET) and the European Carotid Surgery Trial (ECST), and for asymptomatic disease, the ACST (Asymptomatic Carotid Surgery Trial). Note that carotid stenting trials are ongoing at the time of writing.

## Traumatic head injury

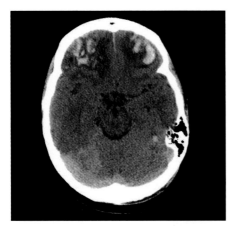

**Figure 5.7**

A 32-year-old woman was involved in a head-on collision (RTA). Her GCS was 11 (E2V4M5) at the scene. On admission to A&E, the patient had a seizure and dropped her GCS to 9/15 (E2V3M4). Her CT head is shown in Figure 5.7.

### Questions

(Q1) What is the diagnosis?

(Q2) Her GCS deteriorates further to 7/15. What should be the immediate management?

(Q3) Explain the concept of cerebral perfusion pressure (CPP).

(Q4) What factors control ICP?

(Q5) Why does hyperventilation decrease ICP at least initially?

(Q6) What surgical interventions can be instituted to regulate ICP?

## Answers

(A1) Bifrontal contusions with significant brain oedema and swelling.

(A2) • ABC and D(isability): thus this patient needs intubation and ventilation to secure her airway, and sedation and paralysis to help control ICP.
• 20–30 degrees of head up.
• Consider mannitol bolus (20%) +/– hypertonic saline.
• iv Benzodiazepines +/– phenytoin/valproate to control seizures.
• Arterial and central venous catheterisation: maintain $P_{CO_2}$ around 4.5 kPa.
• Burr hole/twist drill insertion of either ICP monitor or ventricular catheter with a pressure transducer.
• Consider mild hypothermia.
• Consider inotropes to maintain CPP.

(A3) • CPP = mean arterial pressure (MAP) – ICP, where MAP = 1/3 of pulse pressure + diastolic blood pressure.
• Thus, either decreasing ICP or increasing MAP should increase CPP. This relationship only holds true for brain in which cerebral autoregulation is lost.

(A4) The Munroe Kelly doctrine states that the skull can be considered a closed box containing only three elements; blood, brain and cerebrospinal fluid (CSF). The pressure is related to all three, and in order for equilibrium to be maintained if one is increased, one or both of the others must be decreased to keep the ICP within the physiological range. The simplest example of this is a slow-growing tumour which slowly increases the 'brain' component and displaced CSF until compensation is lost and ICP finally begins to rise.

(A5) Since an increase in $P_{CO_2}$ will cause vasodilation, a decrease will cause vasoconstriction thus decreasing the cerebral blood volume and therefore reducing ICP according to the Munroe Kelly doctrine (above).

(Similar questions could be devised for all factors that can affect ICP, e.g. hydrocephalus involves an increase in the volume of CSF due to either obstruction, over-production or decreased absorption.)

(A6) • External ventricular drainage (to decrease the volume of CSF).
• Decompressive craniectomy (to 'open the box').

# Pituitary tumour

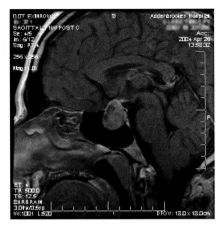

**Figure 5.8**

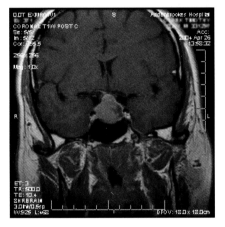

**Figure 5.9**

A 52-year-old woman presents with a history of a number of accidents while driving where 'vehicles just came from nowhere'. A bitemporal visual field defect is picked up at an optician's appointment. On examination the lady has mild papilloedema. Cranial imaging is shown in Figures 5.8 (sagittal) and 5.9 (coronal).

## Questions

**Q1** What is the diagnosis?

**Q2** What can these tumours secrete and what symptoms and syndromes do they produce?

**Q3** What is the aetiology of other effects of these tumours despite those caused by over-secretion of the above hormones?

**Q4** What is the treatment of choice for these tumours?

**Q5** If this patient were to be admitted with confusion, headache and rapidly deteriorating visual fields, what would be the likely diagnosis?

## Answers

 Pituitary tumour – differential:
- macroadenoma (non-secreting vs secreting)
- craniopharyngioma
- meningioma.

- Prolactin (PRL)
  - amenorrhoea–galactorrhoea syndrome (women)
  - impotence (men)
  - infertility (either sex).
- ACTH
  - Cushing's disease.
- Growth hormone (GH)
  - acromegaly in adults
  - gigantism in children (very rare).

 Direct mass effect of the tumour leading to:
- hypopituitarism, hypothyroidism, hypoadrenalism, hypogonadism, diabetes insipidus (rare)
- cavernous sinus pressure and possibly thrombosis: cranial nerve palsies
- pressure on the optic chiasm classically causing a bitemporal field defect as a result of damage to the decussating fibres. Extreme or prolonged pressure can produce blindness.

 Excision by various approaches (trans-sphenoidal/open craniotomy), +/–radiotherapy for any residual left.

**Note**: pituitary hormonal supplementation may be required post-operatively, and electrolytes should be measured daily in the post-operative period.

 Pituitary apoplexy, a neurosurgical emergency requiring immediate decompression. Not an infrequent presentation of a pituitary tumour. This is usually due to an expanding mass within the sella as a result of haemorrhage into the tumour or swelling due to infarction within it.

# Depressed skull fracture

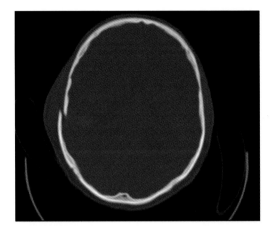

**Figure 5.10**

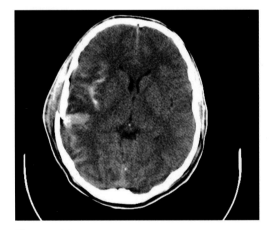

**Figure 5.11**

## Questions

**Q1** What should be the immediate management in A&E?

**Q2** What is the diagnosis?

**Q3** What should be the next priority?

**Q4** What are the criteria for elevation of the flap?

**Q5** Given the contused brain, following lifting of the flap, what further management may the patient require?

A 27-year-old man is assaulted with a baseball bat. He is admitted to A&E with a large laceration on his head, and a GCS of 7 (E2V1M4). His GCS was 12/15 at the scene. Figures 5.10 and 5.11 show CT scans of bone and brain windows at the same level.

## Answers

 • Airway with cervical spine immobilisation, B, C and D(isability).
• The patient is intubated and ventilated for scan.
• A CT scan is performed.

 Depressed skull fracture with underlying contused brain.

 Immediate referral to neurosurgery with a view to lifting the skull flap and debriding the wound.

 • >8–10 mm depression.
• Compound fracture.
• CSF leak, i.e. lacerated dura.
• Deficit related to underlying brain.

 ITU management, ICP pressure control, control of seizures.

# Cauda equina syndrome

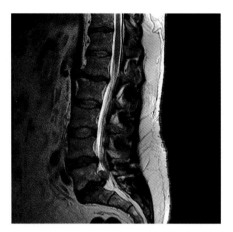

**Figure 5.12**

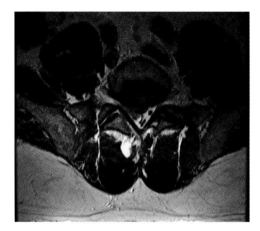

**Figure 5.13**

A 45-year-old builder with a long-standing history of back pain presents with a one-week history of severe bilateral sciatica. He complains when he presents to A&E of a difficulty in passing urine.

## Questions

**Q1** What aspects of the physical examination would be crucial in this case?

**Q2** The findings of the physical examination are sufficiently worrying to organise an urgent MR examination of his lumbosacral spine. This is shown in Figures 5.12 and 5.13. What is the likely diagnosis?

**Q3** What is the immediate management of this patient?

## Answers

(A1) Full neurological examination with particular attention to:
- perianal and perineal sensation: ?'saddle' anaesthesia
- PR: ?anal tone
- +/– insertion of urinary catheter to check for retention and gives an opportunity to ask the patient if they can feel the insertion of the catheter, i.e. do they have normal urethral sensation?

(A2) Cauda equina syndrome secondary to a large, central disc prolapse.

(A3) Immediate neurosurgical/spinal referral for urgent decompressive laminectomy and discectomy. The patient must be warned that he may not get back to normal and many of these patients, if they present too late, either incontinent or in painless retention will need to learn to self-catheterise.

# Subarachnoid haemorrhage

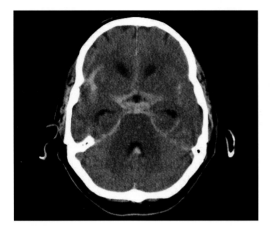

**Figure 5.14**

A 42-year-old migraine sufferer is sitting at the dinner table, when she suddenly grabs her head and complains to her husband of a terrible headache. Feeling nauseous, she retires to bed. The following morning, her husband finds her confused and difficult to rouse. She quickly starts vomiting. On admission to A&E, her GCS is 13/15 (E3V4M6). A CT scan is shown in Figure 5.14.

## Questions

**Q1** What is the diagnosis?

**Q2** What immediate management does this lady require?

**Q3** How could this lady's immediate problem be managed?

**Q4** What further investigation does she require?

**Q5** What are the possible aetiologies of the primary pathology and how could these be managed?

## Answers

- Subarachnoid haemorrhage with blood in the ventricles.
- Hydrocephalus.

 Immediate neurosurgical referral with a view to treatment of the acute hydrocephalus.

 Insertion of an external ventricular drain to relieve the hydrocephalus.

 Imaging of the intracranial vasculature: either formal digital subtraction angiography, CTA or contrast enhanced MRA.

- Aneurysm: surgical clipping or endovascular coiling.
- Arteriovenous malformation (AVM): endovascular embolisation +/– stereotactic radiosurgery +/– open surgery.
- Cavernoma (cavernous haemangioma): endovascular techniques versus open surgery.
- Dural sinus thrombosis: complicated treatment usually involves anticoagulants even in the presence of subarachnoid haemorrhage.
- Rarely tumour.
- Amyloid angiopathy: supportive.
- Vasculitis: treatment of vasculitis.
- Traumatic: usually supportive but dissection of vessels may indicate endovascular intervention.
- Idiopathic.

# Cervical spine fracture

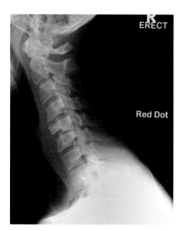

ERECT

Red Dot

**Figure 5.15**

This is the plain lateral radiograph of the cervical spine of a 30-year-old male who fell head-first down some stairs.

## Questions

Q1   What is the abnormality?

Q2   What criteria must be fulfilled to allow the clinician to 'clear' the cervical spine?

Q3   Give examples of a dangerous mechanism of injury.

Q4   What percentage of patients with a cervical spine fracture will have a second spinal injury at another level?

Q5   What is:
- neurogenic shock?
- spinal shock?

## Answers

 There is a wedge compression fracture of C5 with associated soft tissue swelling. There is also loss of the normal cervical lordosis.

- The patient must be fully alert.
- No head injury.
- No neck pain.
- No neurological symptoms nor signs.
- No 'distracting injury'.
- Full pain-free range of movement of neck.

Patients aged under 65 years without a 'dangerous mechanism of injury' who fulfil the above criteria do not require imaging.

- Fall >1 m.
- Fall >5 stairs.
- Axial load to head, e.g. diving.
- High-speed RTA.
- Significant rear end shunt.

 10–15%.

- Neurogenic shock refers to hypotension of neurological origin due to loss of sympathetic vasoconstrictor tone +/– bradycardia. Failure to recognise it may result in fluid overload and pulmonary oedema. It is suggested clinically by hypotension and bradycardia in a patient not on beta-blockers.
- Spinal shock refers to a transient loss of all neurological function below the level of the spinal cord injury resulting in a flaccid paralysis and areflexia.